The Injured Child
An Action Plan for Nurses

The Injured Child
An Action Plan for Nurses

Edited by

Donna M Mead RGN DipN(Lond) RNT RCNT DANS MSc
Senior Research Officer, School of Nursing Studies, University of Wales College
of Medicine

and

J R Sibert MA MD FRCP DCH DObst RCOG
Consultant Paediatrician, Llandough Hospital, South Glamorgan Health
Authority

with eight contributors

SCUTARI PRESS
London

First published 1991

British Library Cataloguing in Publication Data
The injured child.
  1. Children. Injuries
  I. Mead, Donna M.   II. Sibert, J.R.
  617.10083

  ISBN 1-871364-33-7

Typeset by MC Typeset, Gillingham, Kent
Printed and bound in Great Britain by Henry Ling Limited, Dorchester

Contents

Contributors

Janet Bott RGN OND
Formerly Sister, Children's Ward, Manchester Eye Hospital.

Eileen Bottomley RGN RSCN RNT
Formerly Director of Nursing Services, Booth Hall Children's Hospital, Manchester.

Roger Evans FRCP
Consultant in Accident and Emergency Medicine, Cardiff Royal Infirmary.

Anna Foreshaw RSCN
Clinical Nurse Specialist, Thermal Injury, Booth Hall Children's Hospital, Manchester.

Jean Gaffin MSc BSc(Econ)
Secretary, Arthritis Care; formerly Secretary to the Child Accident Prevention Trust and the British Paediatric Association.

Donna M Mead RGN DipN(Lond) RNT RCNT DANS MSc
Senior Research Officer, School of Nursing Studies, University of Wales College of Medicine; Cardiff.

Margaret Morgan RGN RSCN RM RCNT
Clinical Teacher, Neonatal Intensive Care Unit; formerly Sister, Paediatric Accident & Emergency Department, Sheffield Children's Hospital.

J R Sibert MA MD FRCP DCH DObst RCOG
Consultant Paediatrician, Llandough Hospital, South Glamorgan Health Authority.

Julia Walsh RGN RSCN
School Nurse, Surrey District Health Authority.

Frieda M Welch BA RGN RM RHV
Formerly Senior Lecturer in Health Visiting, University of Wales College of Medicine, Cardiff.

Preface

Accidents are the most common cause of death to children after the first year of life and a major cause of handicap and disability. Each year one child in five can expect to attend an Accident and Emergency Department following an accident.

Until recently childhood accidents were regarded as largely unpreventable and their treatment routine, but in recent years the problem has received more of the attention that it warrants. This began with the formation of the Child Accident Prevention Trust and, subsequently, the appearance of several local accident prevention committees. The media then began to pay more attention to the problem, in particular with the *Play it Safe* programmes and, more recently, with a campaign to make travelling by car safer for children.

The King's Fund has recognised the importance of the problem and published *The Management Response to Childhood Accidents* (Constantinides, 1987)—a guide to the effective use of NHS information and resources to prevent accidental injuries in childhood. In 1988 the European Commission launched a crusade against childhood accidents, while the Safety Research Unit of the Department of Trade and Industry, together with the Health Education Authority, supported Pam Laidman's research on the health visitor's role in childhood accident prevention in children under five years of age. Currently the Royal College of Nursing Society of Paediatric Nursing is, in conjunction with the Child Accident Prevention Trust, responding to the challenge of preventing childhood accidents by studying accidents that occur to children while in hospital. That such developments have been effective is reflected in recent successes in childhood accident prevention, including a reduction in accidental poisoning following the introduction of child-resistant containers, a reduction in thermal injuries since the introduction of flameproof nightdresses, and changes in bicycle design resulting in fewer serious injuries following bicycle accidents.

Such success is due to the increasingly high profile that the prevention of childhood accidents is rightly taking. It is fitting that nurses, midwives and health visitors have been involved in many of these developments, because they are ideally placed to play a vital role in the prevention of accidents, either by advising and educating families or by influencing appropriate organisations to make the environment safer for children. Nurses are also ideally placed to ensure that children who have had an accident are cared for in the best possible surroundings.

Given these considerations, it is surprising that there is no nursing text that deals exclusively with the problem of childhood accidents: this book therefore constitutes an attempt to redress the balance.

Child abuse is also an important cause of injury to children. Nurses, midwives and health visitors play an important role in the early detection and management of this problem and are increasingly taking part in the decision-making process for abused children. It was therefore considered that child abuse falls within the remit of this book. However, the problem encompasses much more than just physical injury, and it was thought that little would be gained from separating deliberately induced physical injuries from other forms of child abuse; consequently the relevant chapter attempts to deal with the whole spectrum of child abuse.

This book is written primarily for nurses but will also be of interest and value to those in allied professions. It attempts to address the question of the cause, prevention and treatment of childhood accidents and child abuse. A detailed account of child development is not included because it can be gained from the many excellent texts on this subject. We have, however, attempted to trace the normal stages of development and to identify the types of accident that are likely to occur at different ages. Individual types of accident are considered, as are the general principles of their prevention and management. The nurse's contribution is discussed in a variety of settings, including the community, the Accident and Emergency Department and the hospital ward. We have attempted throughout the book to illustrate how prescribed care and management can be realised in practice, rather than be purely prescriptive—in other words, we have attempted to be descriptive as well as prescriptive.

Donna Mead
J R Sibert

Reference

Constantinides P (1987) *The management response to childhood accidents: A guide to effective use of NHS information and resources to prevent accidental injuries in childhood.* London: Kings Fund.

Acknowledgements

The editors would like to thank a number of people for supporting, criticising and giving practical help during the writing of this book. In particular, we would like to thank Patrick West of Scutari Press, Gill Lyons for her particular contribution to the chapter on child abuse, Mike Hayes of the Child Accident Prevention Trust, Pam Laidman from the Safety Research Unit of the Department of Trade and Industry, and Richard Jones from the Mid Glamorgan School of Nursing. Finally, special thanks go to Jenny Jones and Alison Jenkins for their secretarial support.

DM
JRS

Chapter 1
Introduction to
Childhood Injuries
Donna Mead   J R Sibert

During the past hundred years great improvements have been seen in child morbidity and mortality rates. The control of infection, improved living conditions and better antenatal care have all contributed to a more certain survival. Only 16 in every 1000 children now die in the first year of life, compared with 150 in the early years of this century.

Accidental injury is now the most common cause of death in children over the age of one and constitutes an important cause of death even in children under one year, especially if perinatal deaths are excluded. The Office of Population, Censuses and Surveys (OPCS) reports that 688 children in England and Wales died in 1987 as a result of an accident (Table 1.1), compared with 465 who died from malignant disease. Accidents account for one-third of all deaths of children between the ages of one and 14. Road traffic accidents are the most numerous, but drowning and suffocation, fire and falls are also significant causes of death.

As well as being a common cause of death, childhood accidents are a significant cause of handicap, an important cause of admission to hospital and a frequent cause of attendance at the Accident and Emergency Department. It is estimated that the cost of treating childhood accidents in the UK is more than £180 million per annum. This figure is a reflection of the number of children treated, and is validated by studies in Sheffield and South Glamorgan, which have demonstrated that one child in five will attend hospital because of an accident in any one year. On the basis of such studies it has been estimated that 2.33 million children attend an Accident and Emergency Department annually.

The cost to the NHS and its resources is immense, as are the costs to families. One child from South Glamorgan (Figure 1.1) who is paralysed from the neck down as a result of her injuries is permanently connected to a ventilator and requires constant attention in order to be cared for at home. Alterations and conversions to the family home cost £40,000, and the community nursing team that has been set up to care for her requires an annual budget of £200,000. Her parents have split up since the accident.

Even more alarmingly is the fact that these figures take no account of the accident patients seen by general practitioners. It has been shown that 75 per cent of the children who attend hospital following an accident, for example as a result of a head injury or poisoning, are admitted for observation only.

1

Table 1.1   Fatal accidents, by type, to children 0–14 years in England and Wales, 1987

Type of accident	No. of children killed
Transport Accidents	
Vehicle occupants	80
Pedestrians	214
Pedal cyclists	63
Other	24
Total	381
Home Accidents	
Burns and scalds	89
Suffocation	33
Drowning	20
Falls	11
Poisoning	7
Other causes	37
Total	197
Accidents in other locations	
Drowning	27
Falls	21
Other causes	62
Total	110
Total all accidents	688

Source: OPCS (1988) *Deaths by Accidents and Violence*, Quarterly Monitors DH4 Series.

Nevertheless, it can be seen that 25 per cent of children can expect to receive active treatment.

The real impact of an accident on a child and his family may not be just the initial pain of the injury. Consequences include handicap, and it has been estimated that in England and Wales each year there are 9500 severely and 11 000 moderately disabled children who suffered their injuries through an accident; these figures include those for children brain-damaged from head injuries, drowning and suffocation. The manifestations of handicap can have grave consequences for the child and family, including a new, spoiled identity and adjustment to it – a process sometimes never achieved. Figure 1.2 shows a child who sustained a ruptured spleen, head injuries and a hemiplegia after running into the road in the path of an oncoming car. As well as there being easy access to the road, family psychosocial stress played a part in his accident, as his parents had recently separated. The strain placed upon the family by a severely handicapped child may alter the family dynamics to such an extent that divorce is the only outcome for the parents. There may also be the psychological trauma of a period in hospital for the child or of feelings of guilt for the parents. Finally, the impact of a child's accidental death may leave long-term emotional scars on

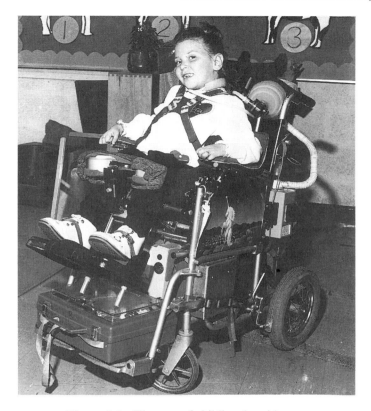

Figure 1.1   The cost of childhood accidents

the family, which can last for a generation.

The OPCS figures so far mentioned are for England and Wales. Similar statistics are found in Western Europe and the United States. It is especially noteworthy that accidental deaths per head of population in children are more common in Third-World countries than in the West, making this an important priority for health care world wide.

In considering the number of children who are injured, the number of deaths, and the impact of the long-term sequelae on the children and their families, it is clear that the problem of childhood accidents is a grave one. Each aspect is worthy of study but until recently has been left largely without research, being looked upon almost as an act of God.

The impact of non-accidental injury is even more difficult to quantify. The very concept that parents might injure their children is not a new one. Kempe (1962) first described the battered-child syndrome and introduced the notion of not accepting parents' explanations for some injuries. It is now recognised that a child may be not only injured non-accidentally, physically, but also neglected or emotionally or sexually abused; indeed, there may be a combination of all these modes of abuse in a single child.

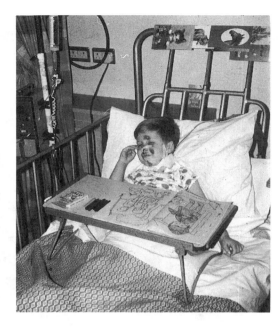

Figure 1.2 A child who suffered a ruptured spleen, head injuries and a hemiplegia after a road traffic accident

How many children die from abuse is really unknown, although estimates have suggested that one child dies each week in England and Wales. The difficulty is that in certain circumstances (for instance suffocation or scalding) the true pattern of events is virtually impossible to determine, and some deaths classified as accidental, may be non-accidental. Similarly, there is evidence that the presentation of non-accidental injury is but the tip of an iceberg in imperfect child care and deprivation. Nevertheless, in a typical area there are 400 substantiated referrals per million inhabitants to the social services each year.

In examining the factors involved in the aetiology of injury to children it is interesting to note that some factors are the same for both accidental and non-accidental injury. There are many social class gradients in both, with working-class children being most likely to be affected. For instance, children of social class V are more than five times more likely to be killed accidentally than those from professional families.

There is also evidence that family psychosocial stress is important aetiologically not only in child abuse but also in accidents. Backett and Johnson (1959) compared a number of families in which a child had been involved in an accident with a control group in which no accident had taken place. Family stress was seen to be more common in the former group. Sibert (1975) found a similar correlation in childhood poisoning. Psychiatric disorder in the mother and other long-standing difficulties such as poor health, shortage of money and marital tension have also been demonstrated as risk factors within the family unit leading to an increased incidence of childhood accidents.

The facts suggest that the borderline between accidental and non-accidental injury may not be a clear one. We may blame the exasperated mother who shakes a child and causes injury to the brain or eye, but should we not also blame the equally exasperated mother who under stress shouts 'Get out of here' and whose child, playing unsupervised, falls from a bedroom window and is equally severely injured?

It has been demonstrated that, for instance, child abuse is more common in families where accidental poisoning had previously occurred (Sibert, 1975). The reason for the heavy social class gradient in accidents is partly environmental, with poor housing and conditions generally being less safe, but is also probably related to more psychosocial stress. The combination of a potentially dangerous environment with a stressful situation is found in many serious accidents in children. A typical case is that of a child with unemployed parents, living in indifferent housing, with easy access for the child to the main road. The child ran out during a birthday party, at which his recently separated parents met in conflict, and sustained a head injury leading to hemiplegia.

Not all aetiological factors are the same in child abuse and accidental injury: more boys are killed accidentally (2.27 : 1) and injured accidentally (1.56 : 1). However, there are no differences in child abuse, apart from those children sexually abused, where girls heavily outnumber boys. The sex differences in accidents are a reflection of the very different behaviour patterns and parental expectations between boys and girls, particularly in play. It would be tempting to say that important differences in behaviour and personality have been shown between accident victims and controls. So-called hyperactivity has perhaps a slight effect on child poisoning and road traffic accidents. However, it is now thought that it is the family circumstances and an unsafe environment that make a child accident-prone rather than an innate problem of behaviour.

One crucial aspect in considering the aetiology of childhood accidents is the age of the child. Children have different accidents at different ages and this is related to child development. Their developmental stage influences the type of accident and also the place where it is likely to occur because children are exposed to different environments as they grow older, although it is often difficult to assess the time spent at home, at school or in the street. The pattern of injuries changes, as does the child's pattern of activities, and for this reason types of injury are discussed under the following categories:

- Infants (birth to 1 year)
- Toddlers (1–3 years)
- Pre-school children (3–4 years)
- School children
- Adolescents

Infants

The child who is under the age of one is totally dependent on his parents for the environment in which he finds himself, and the accidents that occur to this age group are a reflection of this fact. During the first year of life an infant develops the ability to wriggle, roll and shift position, and as he begins to explore his physical environment the learning process involves putting what he finds in his mouth.

The most common cause of injury to infants is falls, normally from one level to another, such as the following:

1.   Falling from a flat surface (30 per cent of injuries to this age group in one study – Jackson et al, 1981).
2.   Falling downstairs – often when being carried by an adult.
3.   Falls occurring when cot sides are left down and the infant is unattended.
4.   Falls when infant seats are left on tables, beds or other furniture.

Other examples of accidents occurring in this age group include:

5.   Those caused by malpositioning of the cot or pram, namely
      (a)   burns, if the cot is placed near a radiator or heating unit;
      (b)   strangulation, if the cot is placed near a window with cords for blinds or curtains, because the infant may become fatally entangled in a dangling cord.
6.   Injuries resulting from the infant sucking a toy, cot side or other object, including those injuries that occur if the paint used on the object contains lead.
7.   Those injuries that result in asphyxiation, such as when button eyes or other small attached parts are pulled off stuffed toys and swallowed by the infant, or when any object small enough to be swallowed is left within his easy reach.
8.   Injuries resulting from leaving an infant unattended with a propped-up feeding bottle.
9.   Suffocation resulting from injudicious use of:
      (a)   plastic-covered mattresses, or pillows;
      (b)   dummies on a long string which can get caught or twisted and result in strangulation;
      (c)   plastic bags, which the infant may put over his head.
10.   Thermal injuries, which may occur if:
      (a)   the temperature of bath water is too high and has not been tested;
      (b)   microwave ovens are used to heat feeds (Puczynski et al, 1983; Sando et al, 1984).

Pre-School Children

Toddlers are adventurous and unpredictable, continually exploring their environment. By the age of three or four they are busily acquiring social skills and attempting to be independent.

The vulnerability of an infant is well recognised, but, as Maddocks (1981) notes, the toddler also needs constant watching and protecting. The phrase 'I need eyes at the back of my head' is often uttered by mothers of this age group. The difficulty of restraining and supervising a toddler while at the same time allowing him the freedom to explore should not be underestimated. He will find any escape route or any potentially dangerous item left unguarded and suitable for exploration.

Many injuries are related to the toddler's eagerness to explore his environment and occur when:

1. he has access to stairways that are not guarded at both head and foot;
2. he has access to unguarded fireplaces or radiators;
3. he is allowed to walk or run while eating, for example, a lollipop;
4. stairs or floors are highly polished or have unfixed rugs.

Injuries may result from the toddler's eagerness to explore specific objects by taking them apart and then putting them back together. This type of accident involves his having access to:

1. sharp objects, such as scissors, screwdrivers or ornaments with sharp edges;
2. matches or lighters;
3. electrical cords;
4. unshielded or unused electric sockets together with objects such as metal knitting needles;
5. unlocked drawers or cupboards that contain anything dangerous.

Injuries can result from the toddler's desire to explore his environment by putting things into his mouth. The following items are particularly dangerous in this regard and should be kept out of his reach:

1. Medicines, disinfectants and household cleaning products.
2. Pins, buttons or needles.
3. Balloons. The child should be closely supervised if he plays with a balloon because aspiration of rubber from broken balloons can be fatal.
4. Foods such as peanuts or popcorn. Again, this is because of the danger of aspiration or asphyxiation.

The toddler's eagerness to explore includes curiosity about things that are higher than eye level. As a consequence, injuries may result from his being able to reach:

1. hot, scalding foods on cookers or work surfaces;
2. handles of pots and pans not protected by a cooker guard or turned towards the back of the stove;
3. tablecloths that hang over the edge of the table;
4. dangling leads of appliances such as irons or toasters.

Climbing is part of the process of exploring, and injuries may result when the toddler climbs onto things. Hazards include:

1. Furniture that is not properly balanced, which may result in the toddler pulling such furniture on top of himself.
2. Windows without properly fitting locks and guards.
3. Car doors that are left unlocked. Also unused refrigerators, freezers and trunks that have not had their doors or locks removed.

Toddlers like to play outside and are fascinated by water. Injuries may occur when:

1. The play area is unfenced and access to the road is allowed;

2. ponds, pools or wells are not fenced or covered. This includes inflatable paddling pools;
3. the toddler is allowed to play outdoors unsupervised, perhaps with older children who may be engaged in rough play;
4. the toddler has not been taught to ride a tricycle on the pavement and to watch for cars in driveways;
5. play equipment such as swings and slides is not properly maintained, either at home or by the local authority.

At pre-school age the child is rapidly gaining independence and confidence in all activities. Maddocks (1981) notes that this is validated by the figures that indicate that there is an increased risk of road accidents and accidents outside the home.

While poisonings become less frequent, episodes of jamming fingers in doors and twisting limbs increase. The safety of the child remains the responsibility of the parents, however, promotion of safety awareness can be initiated in children of this age group. Brunner and Suddarth (1981) suggest that children of this age group can be instructed in the following areas:

1. *Personal Safety*
    (a) To supply information such as their name, address and telephone number.
    (b) To identify firemen, policemen and other safety officials.
    (c) Not to accept a lift or gifts from strangers.

2. *Home Safety*. They can be taught to understand:
    (a) the reasons for various safety measures, such as keeping the floor clear of toys;
    (b) the safe way to use tools;
    (c) kitchen safety;
    (d) the dangers of matches, open flames, hot objects, gas and electrical equipment.

3. *Safety at Play*. Receiving swimming instructions, for example.

4. *Road Safety*. Young children can be taught to understand safety rules and the dangers of traffic.

Schoolchildren

Whereas children between five and seven years have acquired a degree of independence both socially and intellectually, it is accepted that they continue to display unpredictable behaviour. For example, although they will have been informed of the dangers of running out from behind a parked car, given certain circumstances, perhaps a ball rolling out onto the road, they are likely to forget the warning and run onto the road.

It is important to remember that this age group will need to know why precautions are necessary and what the consequences are of failing to follow the rules.

This group of children behaves unpredictably in traffic. Accidents may occur when:

1. the child is not accompanied in traffic – either by a 'lollipop' lady or man or by one of his parents;
2. the child is allowed to play in areas where traffic is not restricted;
3. the child has not been taught the rules of cycling/road safety;
4. the adult road user does not understand the unpredictable behaviour of children in traffic.

Children of this age group are eager to participate in household activities. Injuries can occur as a result of:

1. the child not having been taught the rules of kitchen or garden safety;
2. inappropriate storage of potentially dangerous equipment, for example, kitchen implements, hammers and nails.

A considerable amount of the infant-school-age child's time is spent at home in the house and garden. However, it is children of this age group who are also the major users of parks and playgrounds. Much time is now also spent in playing with other children. The risks of unpredictable behaviour are thought to increase when infant-school children are in a group.

Parents should know of their children's whereabouts at all times. Injuries can occur when they are unsupervised and allowed access to:

1. non-designated play areas such as disused building sites or rubbish dumps, which may contain broken glass, rusty nails, etc;
2. faulty playground equipment that is not regularly inspected and maintained;
3. play equipment that is inappropriate to the child's level of development. The child cannot be expected to decide which roundabout or Jungle Jim is appropriate for him.

Junior-school children aged 7–11 years start to play formal, competitive games, e.g. football, netball and athletics. Development of physical skills occurs and they may become involved in swimming, ballet dancing, gymnastics or cycling. Another characteristic of children of this age group is that they are beginning to become more group-orientated and can often be seen gathered together out of school for informal games. The outcome of group behaviour is uncertain and can lead to aggressive acts.

Accidents may occur as a result of inadequate instruction in relation to outdoor play so that the child is unaware of the dangers of:

1. playing in sandpits;
2. deserted buildings;
3. old refrigerators;
4. playing with fire;
5. playing near railway lines or electricity pylons.

Children of this age group enjoy sport. Accidents may result when:

1. they have not been taught the rules of the sport in which they are involved;

2. they are allowed to use inappropriate or faulty equipment;
3. they are allowed to play competitive games with children older than
    themselves.

Adolescents

Adolescents are the healthiest age group in the population. The commonest
cause of death among this age group is injury – particularly those injuries that
result from a road traffic accident. Avery (1979) estimated that out of every 1000
school-leaving males, approximately 200 will have a road traffic accident
resulting in injury and that three will be killed on the road within 10 years of
leaving school. Over 40 per cent of deaths in males between 15 and 19 are road
deaths, approximately half of which are the result of motor cycle accidents.

Generally speaking, adolescents prefer to be with their peers, to feel part of a
group in which they can try out new ideas, take risks and experiment. They are
becoming increasingly independent and should be encouraged to accept responsibility for their own safety.

Adolescents enjoy the independence that owning their own vehicle, car or
motor cycle, brings. The risk of a road traffic accident occurring increases when:

1. seat belts are not always worn;
2. crash helmets are not worn;   Adolescents resent rules
3. traffic regulations are ignored;   and authority.
4. there is reckless behaviour or
    risk-taking when driving.

Adolescents enjoy taking part in competitive sports. Injuries can result when:

1. as a result of peer-group pressure they attempt to do something that is
    beyond their physical capabilities;
2. dangerous play, especially in rugby football, is not penalised.

Accidents also occur as a result of the adolescent's leisure-time activities.
Rivalry is of great significance in this age group, particularly between boys or
groups of boys. This perhaps explains why 5 per cent of injuries are caused by
fighting.

A knowledge of the injuries sustained by specific age groups is very useful
because target groups can be identified when considering preventive education
programmes. For example, the dangers of scalding from cups and mugs is
almost confined to the first three years of life. The relative risks associated with
each accident type are discussed in the appropriate chapter. The role of the nurse
in child accident prevention is discussed in Chapters 3 and 15.

The Court Report (DHSS, 1976) stated that accidents are the result of the
developmentally immature child encountering a dangerous environment. This
may be because, as Professor Berfestam states, 'We live in an adult world,
designed for adults by adults. It is the responsibility of adults, therefore, to
create an environment which is safe for children to explore.' Court argues that
we should protect the young child and teach the older child to protect himself. It

is important to remember, therefore, that it is the parents who need educating in the first instance. As a child grows older he can be incorporated into such education programmes. The introduction of health education into the school curriculum has played an important part in this – the teaching of road safety, for example, is now a well-recognised part of infant-school life.

If nurses, as health professionals, are to develop efficient and effective teaching programmes, they will need to be able to identify trends in accidents and specific target groups. To this end, nurses need to be prepared to work with epidemiologists, other health care professionals and health educators so that research findings relative to trends and target groups can be communicated and incorporated into effective teaching programmes. Following this, the nurse should be proactive in evaluating education programmes.

References

Avery J G (1979) Motor cycle accidents in teenage males. *Practitioner*, **222**: 369–380.

Backett E M and Johnson A M (1959) Social patterns of road accidents to children. *British Medical Journal*, **1**: 409–413.

Brunner L S and Suddarth D (1981) *The Lippincott Manual of Paediatric Nursing*. London: Harper and Row.

DHSS (1976) *Fit for the Future. Report of the Committee on Child Health Services (Court Report)*. London: HMSO.

Illingworth C M (1977) Paediatric Accident and Emergency Medical or Surgical? *Public Health*, **91**: 147–149.

Jackson R H, Craft A W and Sibert J R (1981) CRC's: the proof of the pudding. *Pharmaceutical Journal*, **226**: 164–165.

Kempe C H, Silverman F, Steele B, Droegmuller W and Silver H (1962) The battered child syndrome. *Journal of the American Medical Association*, **181**: 17.

Maddocks G (1981) Accidents in childhood. *Nursing Mirror*, ii–xiv.

Puczynski M, Rademaker D, Gatson R L (1983) Burn injury related to the improper use of a microwave oven. *Pediatrics*, **72**: 714–715.

Sando W C, Gallaher K J, Rodgers B M (1984) Risk factors for microwave scald injuries in infants. *Journal of Pediatrics*, **105**: 864–867.

Sibert J R (1975) Stress in families of children who have ingested poisons. *British Medical Journal*, **3**: 87.

Sibert J R, Maddocks G B and Brown B M (1981) Childhood Accidents – An endemic of epidemic proportions, *Archives of Diseases in Childhood*, **56**: 225–226.

Recommended Reading

Child Accident Prevention Trust (1989) *Basic Principles of Child Accident Prevention: A Guide to Action*. London: CAPT.
   This excellent publication classifies accidents by types and trends, identifies high-risk groups, explores the issue of who is responsible for prevention of childhood accidents and offers a framework for local and national action.

Gaffin J (1981) Accidents in the home. *Nursing* (1st Series), **23**: 992–994.

Jackson R H (1976) *Children, the Environment and Accidents*. Tunbridge Wells: Pitman Medical.

Wells N (1981) *Accidents in Childhood*. London: OHE Briefing.

Chapter 2
Nursing Management of the Injured Child in the Community
Frieda Welch

Home is ideally a sanctuary – a place of retreat and security, affording confident protection from the hazards of the outside world (Miles, 1972). Houses, however, are designed, built and filled with furnishings and fittings with adults' comforts in mind; they are not designed with child safety as a priority.

First-time parents may have little awareness of the accidents that can occur at home. Nurses, as health educators, can help parents to prevent accidents at home by pointing out the potential hazards: this applies particularly to health visitors, midwives and paediatric nurses, but practice nurses, district nurses and school nurses who have close involvement with families with young children can also help. The role of the nurse working in the community in relation to childhood accidents prevention is discussed later in this chapter.

As we have already seen (Chapter 1), there is seldom a single factor responsible for an accident. It is more likely to be a complex mix of risks associated with human behaviour as well as with the environment, for example, the child who runs out of the house on to a road that is used by heavy traffic, or the depressed mother who leaves her badly packaged tablets on an easily accessible work surface and her child unattended, with the inevitable outcome of accidental poisoning.

It is important that the same risk factors should be taken into account when considering the management of the injured child and his family within the community. Over the past decade great importance and emphasis has been placed on parental involvement in caring for children in paediatric wards. The parent, usually the mother, helps with washing, toileting, feeding and giving minor treatment and medication, and generally stays with the child much, if not all, of the time, when other commitments permit. These activities, however, are carried out within a well-equipped, institutional environment, usually with at least one professionally qualified person helping or supervising and always with somebody within call. A variety of facilities are available: clean dressings can be quickly obtained and soiled ones easily disposed of, a supply of bed linen is to hand, and bedpans, easily accessible toilets and wheelchairs are all items that are taken for granted within a modern ward. Such facilities do not readily exist in the home. However, much credence is given to the idea that the child's own home provides the most advantageous environment for recovery, a belief that is, in part, the result of research undertaken into the effect on the child of separation from his mother (Rutter, 1970; Bowlby, 1969, 1973).

There would appear to be a dearth of research concerning the effects of adverse home circumstances on the recovery of the child. The long-term effects are, regrettably, not always known or recognised by parents and professionals, and objectives are sometimes set which are, with hindsight, unrealistic and unachievable without total subservience of normal family functioning to the need for care. When care demands are such that 'around the clock' attention is necessary, this can and often will impose an intolerable strain on the family unit as a whole and on the mother in particular (Finch and Groves, 1983).

If one compares the hospital setting to the home environment, the actual amount of specialised professional care will perhaps not be radically different. What is different is the pattern of availability, with the hospital providing virtually 24-hour cover, but normal community provision rarely being better than episodic, twice-daily visits, albeit of a significant duration on a one-to-one basis.

When considering the feasibility of managing the injured child at home, the following points should therefore be borne in mind:

1. Whether the child's own home necessarily provides the most advantageous environment for recovery. It can be seen that hospital facilities are not easily or quickly obtained in, or transferred to, a two-bedroomed flat in a multi-storied building or a small, terraced house with less than straightforward access.
2. Whether parents are eager and prepared to provide the care that will be necessary. Eagerness may well exist but the ability to provide care in the full knowledge of what is entailed is another matter.
3. Whether the primary health care team, together with social services, is able to provide a fully comprehensive care programme. For example, recommendations that the primary health care team should be allowed access to central services supplies (CSSD) and to centralised hospital laundry services was made in a 1981 DHSS joint report, but so far its implementation has been patchy.
4. Whether care in the community is a more cost-effective way of using scarce health service resources. The cost in terms of family stress, however, while not comparable in economic terms with hospitalisation, is observably high.

It can be seen that many compromises and much adaptation will have to be made if care of the injured child in the community is to be successfully achieved.

Minor Injuries

The highest proportion of childhood accidents do not involve serious injury. Such children may be seen in the Accident and Emergency Department, where they are treated and then sent home to be cared for by their families. In most instances the parents are advised clearly on how to care for their child and are given instructions to contact the primary health-care team if any further treatment becomes necessary. A letter to their general practitioner, containing details of the injuries incurred and treatment given, is issued.

If communication is good and the family motivated to seek help, an assessment of the particular needs can quickly be made so that the required level of care and treatment can be given. Regrettably, however, there are families who often receive little or no advice and who lack the social skills to recognise and describe their needs, let alone achieve them.

A further group may be given detailed information and instructions about their child's injury and treatment but because of a combination of factors, including an unfamiliar and, to them, threatening environment, the use of clinical terms instead of simple language and inherent social barriers, they incompletely or totally fail to understand or remember this. Such families are often struggling in an adverse environment. It is often the case that they are unable to present the discharge letter to anyone because the health centre or surgery is some distance from the home and there is no-one to look after the child in their absence. The result is that the families most in need of follow-up care receive little if any of it, and where such care is forthcoming it is often only after a long delay.

Problems in relation to ethnicity can further compound the issue. For example, if an injured child from an Asian family requires follow-up care, it is often the case that the mother is not present at the discussions in which advice regarding further management is given. It is usual in such circumstances for the father to be present, and although he may speak English, he may not be given opportunities to explore what the medical and nursing instructions mean. The outcome is that no teaching has been given to the family member, usually the mother, who will be responsible for caring for the child, there is no clear understanding by the family of what criteria to use to decide whether help should be summoned and no clear instructions and arrangements have been given as to the 'how' and 'who' of obtaining help. This, given other social and environmental factors, e.g. racial harassment, could lead to a high-risk situation for a child who may have a moderate condition.

If the injuries have been such that a return visit to the hospital is necessary, this too may present some families with problems. For instance, an injured child may well have to visit more than one hospital department, with a long period of waiting involved each time. In the case of facial injuries this may involve the X-ray Department for follow-up X-rays, the Accident and Emergency Department for the removal of sutures and the surgeon for examination. Such visits require transport, 'respectable' underwear, time (with cover for other family members, e.g. siblings, being essential) and money for transport. Community nursing staff can help with some of these problems. Co-ordination at the hospital or health centre can make all the difference. For example it may be possible to arrange for all departments to be visited on the same day.

Communication links between the Accident and Emergency Department and community staff vary in their effectiveness. As a result of established non-accidental injury procedures, hospital staff are required to inform community health personnel if a child is considered to be 'at risk'. A similar procedure needs to be initiated for children treated in hospital as a result of an accident, as this would enable curative measures to be promoted without delay. With faster referral, services could be mobilised and a better provision for care in the community made available to injured children and their families.

It is also considered essential that the health visitor should visit children who have recently had an accident to offer support and advice on accident prevention, but in order to carry this out, the health visitor needs to be notified of those children who have been treated in hospital following an accident. It is therefore recommended by Laidman (1987) that every district health authority should have a health visitor notification system that covers all hospitals treating children under five years of age. The reader is referred to the section in this chapter on accident prevention and to Laidman (1987) for a detailed account of how such a system should operate.

Serious Injuries

Ideally, before a child with a serious injury is discharged from hospital, a full discussion will have been held by hospital staff (medical, nursing and paramedical), the family (with both parents, if possible) and the primary health-care team. Discussion between the hospital staff, the primary health-care team and, in particular, the paediatric liaison health visitor, will centre on:

1.   the strengths, weaknesses and opportunities of the home environment;
2.   the family's resources;
3.   a full assessment of the child's needs;
4.   the available community resources.

The Home Environment

The World Health Organisation's Report on Community Health Nursing (1974) placed great stress on the role of the family in the provision of care. In our generally affluent society, however, there are many inequalities and imbalances that impinge upon this (Townsend and Davidson, 1982). One of the major inequalities is in the physical or built environment. Generally, children from the Registrar General's Social Classes I, II and III live in favourable neighbourhoods, and their homes are dry, warm, adequately lit and furnished with a degree of space for activity. However, for children from Social Classes IV and V the situation is often far less advantageous. Lack of space, noise, atmospheric pollution and parents with a low income who are therefore unable to indulge in leisure pursuits are only a few of the deprivations experienced. Far too many families live in substandard housing, which is damp, cold, dark and ill-furnished, with little or no free space, and it can be seen that such an environment would not be conducive to promoting the speedy recovery of an injured child.

It is easy to suggest rehousing these families but this is an extremely slow and difficult feat to achieve: for these reasons this is not a feasible solution at this time. Additional, limited financial help can occasionally be obtained from the Departments of Health and Social Security or various charities, but this approach also involves much individual time, travel and effort. Inadequate heating levels constitute a major health hazard but can be alleviated, perhaps by restricting the child to one room (usually the family room, where most normal living activity, which may well include cooking, eating and watching television, occurs). The placing of the child close to his mother has the undoubted advantage that he is less likely to be lonely or bored – and many mothers find this solution less rather than more stressful because the child's demands are fewer, thereby reducing the emotional and physical burden for the mother or caregiver. It presents a difficulty if the child needs rest, but many children will sleep soundly in the midst of a high level of surrounding noise and activity.

Achieving and maintaining an acceptable standard of hygiene is possible with discipline and ingenuity even for families in adverse housing conditions, but it does depend on the individual child's circumstances.

Child Profile

Age is an important consideration, with critical developmental stages of particular relevance because of the differentiation of approach and management that may be necessary. It can be seen, for example, that the child's level of maturation and intellectual and educational development will influence his ability to participate in and respond to treatment. Such factors are also an important ingredient in the psychological contract that exists under such circumstances between the child, the family and outside agencies.

The child's physical make-up is also an important variable in the care equation, with such factors as motor skills and mobility levels being important considerations. The sex of the child may also influence behaviour, although this will depend greatly upon the social mores. However it is likely that a child will have been socialised into developing behaviour patterns that are appropriate to his or her sex, for example aggressive, active boys and docile, gentle girls.

The child's position within the family will affect the parents' capacity to meet needs and apportion resources. An only child, for example, can become the focus for excessive parental care. Where this occurs anxiety leading to neurosis, often to the extent that it is detrimental to re-establishing the child's independence, may be displayed.

A child from a larger family may have to compete for attention with siblings, older, younger or both. In addition, the injured child may well have to be protected from the attention of a bossy older sister or a boisterous younger brother, not to mention an exuberant family dog!

The nature of the child's injuries is one of the most important considerations when making the assessment. The amount of time that will need to be invested should be considered alongside the parents' capacity to provide it and the resources in the community to support the parents in this endeavour.

Community Resources

Faith in the ability of the primary health-care team, together with the community social services, to provide a fully comprehensive care programme is often ill-founded, especially when families in unfavourable circumstances are involved. In terms of resources, the local authority social services department can often supply cots and beds, and blankets and clothes can be obtained from such sources as the WRVS, the Red Cross and the Salvation Army. Prudent clinic or health-centre staff will take every opportunity to utilise the material resources of any favourably disposed organisation in their locality.

Staff must be realistic in deciding whether or not community provision in terms of both manpower and resources is sufficient to meet the needs of the injured child. It must be remembered that it is the family that will provide the care, with intervention only coming from the primary health care team. This is why the family profile is one of the most important considerations in deciding the feasibility of returning the injured child to be managed in his own home.

The Family

A serious or potentially serious injury to a child often produces a physical and emotional crisis within the family unit. If the environment is stable and support systems are available and adequate, many families are able to adapt to the situation and contain it. However, where the family unit is less stable or inadequately supported, additional input from various agencies may well be essential to stabilise the situation.

There is often a variety of feelings within the family following an injury to a child, which include shock, fear, anger and guilt. As a result some parents display a severe loss of confidence in themselves and in their parenting skills. Alternatively, anxious parents may think that they have been found lacking and overcompensate in their effort to mitigate the effects. It is absolutely essential that the primary health-care worker should be alert to this fact when making an assessment of the family's ability to care for the injured child. If adequate parenting skills have previously been apparent and if the emotional climate was warm and secure before the event, there is every reason to believe that after the initial shock has subsided things will again stabilise and the parents' confidence in themselves will be restored. For the less fortunate child whose emotional environment lacks equilibrium, the trauma can be a contributory factor in a further destabilising process.

In making an assessment of a family's ability to cope with an injured child at home the parents' age, social status and values will need to be considered, as these are important determinants for the establishment of expectations and objectives, and their realisation by appropriate strategies. Educated and articulate parents will harness the system to their advantage and often display a level of knowledge and applied skills equal or superior to many professional staff. With such capabilities they can usually achieve their needs with minimal assistance and maximum effectiveness.

The less advantaged parents who, perhaps, may be unable or unwilling to make a positive entry into the system are much more vulnerable and it is for such families that positive discrimination may well be appropriate and necessary.

A very real advantage of working as a health visitor or community nurse lies in having a unique knowledge of families with children: this often means that a good working relationship has already been established. This knowledge provides a sound basis from which to assess the family's ability to cope with an additional crisis. A mother who recognises when her child is ill enough to require medical attention and seeks it promptly will almost certainly behave in a like manner. A family unit that has functioned effectively over a period of time, met and contained other crises for example childbirth, bereavement and unemployment, is likely to adapt to a new situation and remain a stable unit. The nuclear family without extended family support available or easily accessible can be more at risk. If interaction with neighbours is good, however, this can provide a valuable source of surrogate mechanisms.

One family in eight is a single-parent family. Such families often receive excellent back-up from their extended families and, in addition, much support is given by various voluntary agencies such as Gingerbread.

The family who is at odds with the world, however, is very vulnerable indeed. Relationships with neighbours are often bad, and the general practitioner and health visitor may be changed so frequently that there is little or no continuity of care. It may also be that the family is attached to a poor, inaccessible, inner city GP practice. Families with this sort of background tend to take the child to the Accident and Emergency Department for even the most basic of health problems, often travelling to different hospitals in rotation. Conversely, such families may not seek medical help at all. Home management skills are low in families with this sort of profile and it is often the case that the social services will be involved with them. In addition, there may be a history of violence, and the police, school welfare or probation department may also be visiting. It may well be a very difficult decision to make, but this could be too adverse an environment for an injured child to return to or remain in. A case conference involving health and social work staff may be necessary, for this child could be at risk also of non-accidental injury.

It is essential for the maintenance of good relationships and provision of care that the parents are involved in this process of evaluation. Their feelings and fears are important considerations. Their knowledge base must be established and, if low, a remedial programme may need to be implemented. Where possible, their coping capacity as a family may have to be assessed. In the case of an injured child this would be levelled at the family's ability to deal with health problems with reasonable success. Freeman and Heinrich (1981) define six health tasks for the family:

1. Recognising interruption of health or development.
2. Seeking health care.
3. Managing health and non-health crises.
4. Providing nursing care to sick, disabled or dependent members of the family.
5. Maintaining a home environment conducive to good health and personal development.

6. Maintaining a reciprocal relationship with the community and its health institutions.

These health tasks provide a useful tool with which to assess the parents' competence to manage an injured child at home. In conjunction with the physical and social assessment, the family's ability to perform these tasks can provide a basis for the evaluation of parental competence and motivation. Following such an assessment, the family's ability to deal with the injured child at home would then be rated upon a referential scale, such as the following, suggested by Freeman and Heinrich (1981):

1 point. No competence, needing high intervention.

3 points. Moderate competence, regular intervention until level raised.

5 points. Complete competence, surveillance and reinforcement intervention only.

To achieve a high level of replicable comparability, such scoring demands careful training and standardisation approaches to produce the skills level needed. However, the importance of such an evaluation is that it enables the level of nursing intervention required to be established and tailored to fit the specific needs of the family. This would then be followed by implementation of the plan of action and continuous monitoring of progress.

Any care plan must have clearly discerned, simply specified, realistically achievable objectives. Parents must be willing and able to carry out the activities decided upon. The best use should be made of available material and human resources. A means for assessing progress and varying strategies to meet developing needs must be employed, and a calendar for action when preparing the care plan might include the following appraisal stages:

- *Interim*   How best to react now; containment.
- *Adaptive*   Improvement and further adaptation.
- *Corrective*   Modify environment, remove cause, treat effect.
- *Preventive*   Be prepared, educate and communicate.
- *Contingency*   Avoid surprises, plan ahead, update and disseminate.

Sample: 24-hour programme overview

Assessment

Child   Five-year-old male. Severe facial bruising with sutured laceration of chin.
                   Reluctant to co-operate.
Family   Mother.
                   Father, working night shift.
                   Two other, younger children.
Home environment   Two-bedroomed flat; toilet and washing facilities adequate.

Care Objectives

A well-hydrated child (fluid intake and liquid nourishment 2–3 litres within 24 hours).
Acceptable level of pain containment (3-hourly analgesia).
Low level of activity (partial bed rest).
Wound remains clean, dry, uninfected.

Possible Strategies (creating alternatives)

Child   Persuasion/coercion/bribery.
        Baby feeders/bottles/bendy straws.
        Iced fluids/minerals/flavoured drinks.
        Medication/tablet/syrup/crushed.
Family Use of grandparents/neighbours/others.
        Day nursery/nursery school/crèche.
        Nursing/health visitor intervention.

Selection of the Best (feasible rather than possible)

Father lodges next door. Neighbour lives in or boards younger children and mother is able to give exclusive time and attention between catnaps for 48 hours (less if swelling subsides). Community nurse/health visitor calls morning and evening, if considered necessary, to give advice and any practical assistance required.

Teaching Input

Primarily dependent upon the nature and assessment of injury and parental competence.

Fluid intake needs	Explain rationale – reinforce, discuss. Demonstrate techniques that may be used to ensure the child receives the required intake.	
Medication	Discuss administration with regard to the child's general condition. Clarify dosages and frequency with maxima clearly understood. Consider alternating methods of administration.	Through stories or quiet play ensure the child understands the importance of co-operating.
Activity level	Discuss ways and means of restricting activity and maintaining a high level of surveillance.	
Care of wound	Observation and cleansing of the wound area Discuss advantages/disadvantages of dressings/open exposure.	

It can be seen that it is vitally important when planning a care programme for the injured child and his family that known risk factors are identified, understood and accepted by the family and health-care professionals. This open acknowledgement will enable a realistic threshold to be established for the minimum level of care essential for the child's recovery and the necessary support to be given to the child and family to achieve this.

It is to be hoped that such an endeavour will also raise consciousness to the possibility of re-occurrence of the accident so that preventive measures can be initiated.

The level of required medical input would be established and the paediatric health visitor and/or community nurse, together with the ward nursing staff and parents, would agree the threshold level needs of the programme. Objectives that are fully subscribed to and understood by all parties concerned are clearly spelt out. Direct channels of communication must be established with specific names, addresses, telephone numbers and contact times given. In addition, adequate strategies to enable both the parents and the health professionals to cope with a range of possible problems should be decided upon. This may be considered to be a counsel of perfection but it is necessary if parents are to be considered adequately prepared for their task.

It is often the case that there are no easy solutions and only limited options when planning to manage the injured child at home. When the physical environment is such that it would actively endanger the child's recovery or when the parents' coping index is unfavourable, one such option may include the child remaining in hospital until he is fit enough to function normally. Where available, respite care provides excellent support for the family, in extreme circumstances it may be necessary to arrange temporary foster care.

The Role of the Health Visitor in Child Accident Prevention

This section is largely based on the work of Laidman (1987) *The Health Visitor's Role in the Prevention of Accidents to Children Between Antenatal and Pre-school Age*. Any nurse interested in the prevention of childhood accidents is strongly advised to read this research report, which examines the problems faced by health visitors in the field and outlines realistic and practical recommendations to improve the service. Laidman points out that it is inevitable that any piece of work that examines a service with a view to improving it will appear critical, and she stresses that the research offers no criticism of the health visiting profession. Its aim is to support health visitors in overcoming the constraints and limitations placed upon them, as these reduce their effectiveness in child accident prevention.

There is evidence that suggests that the impact on individual families of short- and long-term publicity campaigns, e.g. the *Play it Safe* booklet, is limited and that an integrated, sustained level of contact is required if children's home safety is to be promoted. It is also known that advising an individual on a one-to-one basis at the site of the hazard is more likely to achieve a positive result than a distant or group approach (Colver et al, 1982).

In practical terms, health visitors are likely to be the most appropriate intermediaries to promote accident prevention within the home. In fact, Laidman (1987) argues that the health visitors' specialist communication skills and their preventive mode of working sets them apart from other professionals in this respect. Their community base and detailed knowledge of their clients, the neighbourhood and local facilities gives them a sound foundation upon which to build a role in child accident prevention.

Such a role is seen as one of their areas of responsibility, and with their knowledge health visitors can identify priorities between different accident types and also the most effective way of presenting the necessary information. Health visitors have repeated contact with families containing young children; indeed, they are the only professional group to visit all such families and thus have the access to parents that no other group enjoys. They meet their clients at clinics and at group sessions and (most importantly) they also are invited into clients' homes. Thus they have a one-to-one contact with clients at the site of a potential accident. The health visitor's repeated visits to clients' homes in accordance with a developmental timetable enables them to give a series of safety messages in a structured sequence. This increases the number of safety topics that can be covered and also allows for repetition and reinforcement of messages and for reward when action is taken.

The aims of such safety education should be to change attitudes towards safety, to increase awareness of the causes of potential accidents, their effect and their prevention, and to encourage a change in behaviour that results in a safer environment and thereby achieves, in the long term, a reduction in accidental mortality and morbidity.

Laidman (1987) notes that one of the most important issues to bear in mind when planning a programme of safety education is targeting. This includes targeting both the topic and the audience. We know from educational research that if too much information or too general a message is given, the effectiveness of the programme will be reduced. The health visitor should address only one or two specific topics at a time to ensure that the families concerned have an opportunity to understand the messages and take them on board. It is often the case that advice about accidents is combined with a variety of other advice about child care, and when this occurs the advice about accident prevention is likely to be missed – either because too much information was presented or because it was not seen to be important when compared with, for example, advice about the child's feeding patterns.

Colver et al (1982) found that even severely disadvantaged families will respond to health education if the education is appropriate. Of families who were given specific advice about hazards present in their homes at the time of the home visit, 60 per cent instigated at least one change to make their homes safer.

With any type of accident there are certain groups of the population who are likely to be most at risk. Indeed, for any individual the accident hazards present will be unique in terms of the risk and the relative priority given to each. The hazards will also alter over time if there is a growing child in the household. In general, to ensure that the time, effort and money available are put to best use, selected target topics should be covered with a selected target group of the population who are most at risk of the particular accident. In an ideal world, each individual needs and should be supplied with a specifically tailored safety programme.

Laidman (1987) further notes that the target topic and the selected, contactable audience are only the start of planning a safety education programme. A decision must also be made as to the best way in which to present a message. The advantages of advising an individual on a one-to-one basis at the site of the hazard have already been noted as having a more positive result than distant or group approaches. Often a series of techniques may be used within a single programme. Whichever method of presentation is used, it is important that the messages are presented in such a way that the audience is as actively involved as possible. For example, leaflets should be looked at together and not just left, and films should be discussed and not just watched. It should also be noted that some methods of presenting information are inappropriate for some audiences; for example, the use of detailed, written information is more appropriate for middle-class groups.

The content of each message should also be given careful consideration, and several factors are important. First, the message must be relevant to the audience selected. It is pointless to talk about safety glazing to a council tenant – it would be more appropriate to discuss such a matter with the council itself. Second, the message should relate to the environment, facilities and situation of the audience and should include local information and local examples wherever possible. Third, it is important that the message should not only detail a dangerous situation but also identify and promote practical measures for accident prevention that are within the power of the audience to implement.

It can be seen that, in theory, the health visitor is in an ideal position to carry out an effective role in child accident prevention. She has the opportunity to visit people, the knowledge to offer and the skills to communicate the information. Laidman (1987), however, also found that while in theory child accident prevention is given a fairly high priority, in practice its level of importance is flexible and is often overtaken by the perceived needs of the client. This is compounded by the fact that parents are unlikely to ask about safety even though the health visitor is seen by them as a potential source of advice. Laidman suggested that patients satisfy their own (possibly inappropriate or unreliable) basic set of safety criteria and thus consider their child to be as safe as is possible or desirable. This not only leaves the onus upon the health visitor to introduce the subject but also erects attitudinal barriers against any advice given.

During the course of Laidman's (1987) research the constraints placed upon health visitors that reduce the effectiveness of the health visitor's role in child accident prevention were collated. The problems that were identified by health visitors fall into three main categories.

Knowledge

The relative priority given by health visitors to child accident prevention over other topics covered is considered appropriate. Furthermore, many health visitors were found to be quite aware of the most appropriate ways to deliver preventive education. The accident-prevention information made available to health visitors through initial training, in-service training and local resources was often found to be limited. Local safety resources and facilities are not collated and many health visitors rely on the often-distorted presentations of the media. In addition, there are only a limited number of safety materials available to the health visitor at present.

It became evident as a result of Laidman's research that there are only a limited number of new publications that facilitate the health visitor's role in child accident prevention, the most popular of which is *Play it Safe*. However, an omission in this booklet resulting from its arrangement of accidents by type is a comment on the relationship between accidents and child development. In any publication on safety it would be useful if a section were included that identified and explained the link between accidents and child development (physical, cognitive and emotional) and encouraged anticipatory, preventive action.

Laidman (1987) argues that no matter how good *Play it Safe* is perceived to be, its one big drawback is that it can be utilised by the health visitor only so many times with a particular family before it loses its impact: there are occasions when other material is needed to reinforce the message. In addition, certain clients and safety topics need specific support material; such as the recently produced booklet *Keep Them Safe* (Child Accident Prevention Trust, 1986/7), an illustrated guide to child safety equipment. It is recommended that this type of booklet, which contains very specific information, is produced to supplement any major-accident prevention booklet. In addition, it is recommended that a series of single-sheet leaflets be produced, each explaining a stage in a child's development, the hazardous situations the child faces and suitable preventive measures. This series of leaflets is envisaged as a simple affair that the health visitor could use with parents. The information they would contain would be brief and to the point, and space would be left for the addition of local information. The leaflets would act as a reminder to health visitors as well as to their clients.

In addition to leaflets, the health visitors in Laidman's study identified the need for new posters and other visual aids appropriate to local needs. For example, in areas in which there are high-rise flats, posters displaying the need for window locks would be useful. It is recommended that posters and other material for display at clinics or to groups should be developed in collaboration with health visitors and their clients at a local as well as national level.

Opportunity

The opportunities for repeated, direct, one-to-one contact within the home with all parents of young children often do not, in reality, exist. Case-load sizes, the pressure of other priorities and an increase in crisis visiting can all reduce the opportunities for safety education. Such a situation reduces the preventive, anticipatory nature of the health visitor's role to that of a reactive, social-work nature.

The main reason found for the reduced visiting schedule was a lack of health visitors. Such a situation may be the result of posts being left unfilled, insufficient trainees being employed to replace those leaving the profession, or an inadequate quota of health visitors being set in the health district. This was most apparent in many deprived, inner-city health districts. The result of insufficient health visitors was found to be very large case-loads for those who were employed. The size of case-loads can lead to a reduction in visiting, especially at the key ages when a child is most at risk of an accident. The use of the clinic to cover these ages is inappropriate, in part owing to the low attendances, but also because those who do attend are probably those least in need of safety education and because it has been shown that the clinic is not as effective in giving individual advice as a health visitor on a home visit.

It has also been shown that people from the lower socioeconomic groups and those under stress from a variety of deprivation and social factors have children who are most likely to have an accident (Townsend and Davidson, 1982). These are the people most in the need of the information, advice and support that the health visitor can offer. Through Laidman's study it has become apparent that these families are often those who are offered least by health visiting services. No matter how good is the individual health visitor, the full extent of health visiting cannot be met if the case-load size does not reflect the needs of the area. 'Problem' areas should have smaller case-load sizes than the norm, not larger, to allow the full effectiveness of the health visitor's role in child accident prevention and other topics to be realised.

Skills

Given suitable opportunities and sufficient and appropriate knowledge, health visitors also need the skills to have an effective role in child accident prevention. Health visitors are among the best trained and most able community workers; in particular, they have well-developed communication skills. The ability to communicate advice to a client effectively is the keystone of safety education.

The health visitor–client relationship is at the centre of good-quality health visiting practice. If this relationship is good, advice can be more direct and working with a client is reported to be easier, but without such a relationship communication can become difficult. For example, it was usually considered inappropriate to mention accident prevention during the first few home visits, as many of the points that need to be made stress things that the parents have not seen and/or have not done, and are therefore critical of their parenting skills and of the level of care they give their child. Various strategies were identified by which health visitors try to overcome these problems, such as slipping safety into a discussion of another topic or talking around the subject. However, such strategies serve to diminish the importance of accident prevention as a topic in its own right and to fragment safety messages into isolated, dangerous scenarios rather than the desired conceptual framework upon which a client could decide on further action. The impact of the health visitor's safety education role is therefore reduced. New communication approaches need to be developed and a new balance drawn between effective safety education and the need for a positive approach. The importance of the health visitor–client relationship should not be overlooked; it is possible to develop a range of communication strategies to ensure that accident prevention is specifically dealt with while existing relationships are preserved.

It is recommended that within initial and in-service health training a significant proportion of the time available be used to develop safety communication skills. This is not meant to imply that safety needs different communication skills from other topics within the health visitor's remit, but rather that the communication skills need to be finely tuned to deal with safety. In particular, the courses should concentrate on the skills needed to initiate a discussion on accident prevention and to continue it to a successful end. The difficulties of offering safety advice to clients who are under stress from a variety of problems and during a post-accident visit should be highlighted. It is felt that this preparation for safety skills teaching is most important during initial training. The students need to be able to discuss the problems and difficulties they may face in the field and to practise a variety of approaches.

With an improvement in their knowledge and refinement of their skills, health visitors can make the most efficient and effective use of the time available to them to carry out their safety education role.

One other area of concern that should be mentioned here is that of accident notification procedures and resulting post-accident visits. It is considered essential to the health visitor's role in accident prevention that she should visit children who have recently had an accident to offer support and preventive advice. To carry out this role she needs to be notified of all children from her case-load who have been treated in hospital following an accident. Therefore, it is recommended that all district health authorities have a health visitor notification system that covers all hospitals treating children under five years of age. To be effective these systems have to fulfil certain criteria. It is suggested that district health authorities with a notification scheme should initiate an evaluation of the speed of the service and establish and implement improvements where appropriate. In addition, it is recommended that health visitors be notified of all child accident cases regardless of their route into hospital. Thus wards, clinics and the Accident and Emergency Department will all be involved.

It is not anticipated that every case will receive a post-accident visit from a health visitor, but the field health visitor is in the best position to decide when a visit is appropriate. Thus no pre-notification selection criteria should be operated within the hospital.

Finally, for a notification system to be efficient it must supply the information that is needed. A basic data set can be identified that includes the child's name and address, date of birth, GP's name, dates of arrival and discharge, injury received, treatment given, cause of injury and future action. In addition, it is suggested that information is supplied about recent hospital contacts, especially a history of previous accidents, on whether the client was advised that a health visitor may call and whether the hospital staff considered at any time that the injury may not have been accidental. This information can be invaluable to the health visitor when deciding on whether or not a post-accident visit is required.

As a result of Laidman's research a series of recommendations with practical implications has been outlined. It is hoped that two major recommendations for improvement will be realised. First, an increase in the quantity and quality of information on child accident prevention should be available for initial and in-service training. This should include a 'communication skills for safety' component and supply a conceptual framework for future work. Second, guidance should be given on the selection of priorities with regard to accident prevention to help the health visitor select the most appropriate advice to give in different visiting situations. This does not imply an attempt to dictate to health visitors how they should act: they are better placed to decide on the position and needs of their clients. However, it should supply the facilities and background upon which to base local preventive decisions (see Laidman 1987 for proposed strategies for guidelines).

In conclusion, Laidman notes that health visitors are, or should be, the primary workers, the leaders of action, in community health, who can spearhead local preventive programmes on a variety of subjects. Within the field of child accident prevention it is possible that they could exercise their full role and directly influence both the safety behaviour of their clients and their colleagues in other professions. Health visitors can help to prevent accidents to the pre-school child.

References

Bowlby J (1969) *Attachment and Loss, I: Attachment.* London: Hogarth Press.

Bowlby J (1973) *Attachment and Loss, II: Separation, Anxiety and Anger.* London: Hogarth Press.

Child Accident Prevention Trust (1986/7) *Keep Them Safe: A Guide to Child Safety Equipment.* London: Child Accident Prevention Trust.

Colver A F, Hutchinson P J and Judson E C (1982) Promoting children's home safety. *British Medical Journal,* **285**: 1177–1180.

DHSS (1981) *Report of the Joint Working Committee of the Standing Medical Advisory Team and the Standing Nursing and Midwifery Advisory Committee* (The Harding Report). London: DHSS.

Finch J and Groves D (1983) *A Labour of Love: Women, Work and Caring.* London: Routledge and Kegan Paul.

Freeman R B and Heinrich J (1981) *Community Health Nursing Practice.* London: W B Saunders.

Health Education Council and the Scottish Health Education Group, in association with the BBC (1981) *Play it Safe: A Guide to Preventing Children's Accidents.* London: HEC/SHEG.

Laidman P (1987) *The Health Visitor's Role in the Prevention of Accidents to Children between Antenatal and Pre-school Age.* London: Health Education Authority.

Miles S (1972) Foreword to *Medical Aspects of Home Hazards.* London: The Medical Commission on Accident Prevention.

Rutter M (1970) *Maternal Deprivation Reassessed.* Harmondsworth: Penguin.

Townsend P and Davidson N (1982) *Inequalities in Health: The Black Report.* Harmondsworth: Penguin.

World Health Organisation (1974) Expert Committee on Community Health Nursing. *Technical Reports Series,* **558**: 10–12. Geneva: World Health Organisation.

Resources

Child Accident Prevention Trust
75 Portland Place
London W1N 3AL

Royal Society for the Prevention of Accidents
Cannon House
The Priory
Queensway
Birmingham B4 6BS

Chapter 3
Nursing Management of the Injured Child in the Accident and Emergency Department

Margaret Morgan

It is important that after an accident children should be treated in the best possible environment and that if that environment is an Accident and Emergency Department it should be as 'unhostile' as possible. The first impressions of the department are important, for even if the child is badly injured, his surroundings can have an effect – especially if he is in a young age group. Decor and layout should be bright and welcoming. Wallpaper, posters and curtains with familiar figures – television, book or nursery-rhyme characters – help to make the department less hostile. Pictures or posters on the ceiling will distract a child who is lying flat on a trolley.

If children are treated in a general Accident and Emergency Department, a separate area should be created for them with suitable decor and furniture. Such an area can be provided at most Accident and Emergency Departments at low cost (Richmond et al, 1987). Adult-sized chairs, tables and trolleys will dominate and frighten the child more than scaled-down versions. Being surrounded by ill, injured and often aggressive adults will also frighten the child.

Plenty of toys and books should be provided to entertain the child during the often long wait and to act as distractions during examination or treatment. Opportunity should be given for play: a separate room is the ideal, but where this is impossible an area in the department should be set aside for this purpose. Oakshot (1973) points out that play is one of the ways of absorbing stress and emphasises the importance of provision for play in hospitals. Of particular concern is the young child who, argues Oakshot, has no other means of communication. Many people are willing to donate toys and books if they know that such items are needed.

The different areas of the department should be clearly defined and marked, as people in distress or panic are easily confused. All parts should be easily accessible, particularly the resuscitation area. The entrances for emergency patients and ambulant patients should be separate. The waiting area should be clearly marked and the waiting systems explained fully.

Staff

Both pleasant surroundings and the right staff are essential to the creation of an environment conducive to the care of the injured or ill child. An understanding of the normal development and behaviour of all age ranges is essential in assessing the reaction of the patient. Senior nurses caring for children in the Accident and Emergency Department should have paediatric nursing qualifications.

Equipment

A range of small instruments and other specific paediatric equipment, in particular paediatric resuscitation equipment, should be available. Formulations of commonly needed drugs for children should also be easily accessible.

Medical Records

Note-keeping in the Accident and Emergency Department is extremely important. The transient nature of the patients, the number of different disciplines dealing with them and the medicolegal implications make accurate recording of personal and social details and treatment essential. The format of the accident and emergency forms for recording all information can ensure that sufficient personal and accident details are noted, but medical and nursing staff should ensure that they record, in full, all details of examinations performed, including negative as well as positive findings, and the treatment and care given.

All past notes for the same patient should be kept together and the index system upgraded and cross-referenced as necessary. In this way regular accident or illness patterns can be noted. For example, unusual fractures may suggest child abuse, which may be missed if each attendance is taken in isolation.

Information recorded on admission should include: name and address, GP and health visitor, date and time of admission, date and time of accident or illness, location of accident and whether or not it was reported to the police. Knowing whether the child was a pedestrian, on a bicycle or a passenger in a car may also be useful. The names of the doctor and nurse attending the child on each visit should also be noted.

The computerisation of accident and emergency records was recommended by the Korner Committee (Steering Group on Health Services Information, 1982). This would have important advantages for children – noting accident trends among susceptible groups, detecting children at risk and making the transfer of information to nurses and doctors in the community easier. Widespread use of computerised Accident and Emergency Department records is still awaited.

Initial Assessment: Priorities and Approaches

Assessment of the severity of the child's condition and the need for immediate treatment is vital in the management of patients and resources in the Accident and Emergency Department. It is now accepted that such sorting of patients in order of priority, or triage, is best done by an experienced nurse. In an Accident and Emergency Department that receives children, experienced paediatric nurses should be available for this purpose. In general, children are usually given priority over other admissions except where severe injuries are involved. The nurse should assess the child's condition and give emergency treatment while waiting for the doctor, if necessary asking the doctor to attend immediately.

In general, those emergencies that are the result of an accident and which require immediate treatment include:

- unconsciousness;
- major accidents;
- burns and scalds;
- all eye injuries;
- compound and simple displaced fractures;
- ingestion of poisons;
- head injuries when the child displays drowsiness, vomiting, unusual behaviour or convulsions;
- severe lacerations;
- finger-tip injuries.

The Approach to the Child

It is important to remember that the child should be approached correctly and given adequate and appropriate instructions and explanations. Much time and effort can be saved by gaining the child's co-operation and trust from the outset. There are many ways of achieving this and obviously each child is an individual, but by trying to understand his reactions and feelings the nurse will be in a better position to support him and his family.

Dealing with the Child Under Stress

The injured child may be frightened or overwhelmed after the accident by the strange environment of the Accident and Emergency Department, with its strange people, noise and bustle, and by his frightened parents. He may react by being unco-operative and unreasonable from the outset, or be silent but equally unco-operative when approached by anyone other than his parents.

Immediate examination and undressing for other than major injury is not desirable because it can cause emotional problems for the child. A steady flow of talk, with distracting toys for the smaller children or explanations for older children can help to reassure and calm the child before any examination is attempted. Involving the parents in care from the outset by getting them to assist in this early stage will help to calm them, too.

Babies and very young children (0–2 year olds) will not be able to understand explanations. Distracting toys combined with swift execution of the examination and treatment are the best way of dealing with these children. When attempting a difficult examination it is easier if the act is made into a game. For example, attempting to examine the fundus of the eye may only be possible if the young child is allowed to play with the ophthalmoscope and follow the magic light over his body until it reaches the eye, then watch it until you blow it out.

Toddlers should be given simple explanations. All information given must be honest. If a child is told that a procedure will not hurt when it does, his trust in the staff will have been lost: subsequent treatment and return visits will then be more traumatic for everyone. Dolls and teddy bears can be used as role models to demonstrate what the nurse is about to do to the child. For the school-age child, adequate explanations are essential. Hyson (1983) observed that crying often occurs in anticipation of harm rather than from the actual procedure. It follows that by explaining everything that is happening, or is about to happen, the child will not anticipate imagined harm. If possible, continuity of staff should be maintained throughout the child's stay in the department. This helps the child to form a brief attachment and also gives staff satisfaction.

Approach to the Family

It should be remembered that parents of very young children often need more reassurance than does the child. Guilt that the accident occurred while the child was in their care, the feeling that they have not met their responsibilities and one member of the family being blamed by another can all produce an emotional reaction that may be directed at the nearest person, usually the nurse or the doctor, in the form of aggression or complaint.

A calm, sympathetic approach is necessary, with a brief explanation of the nature of the injury and treatment that will be given. Reassurance should also be given, if possible, and can help to calm the parents. For example, the information that no scarring will result from a superficial burn will help to allay guilt, and that a profusely bleeding scalp wound is, in fact, quite small, will disperse fears of serious head injury.

Obviously such optimistic outcomes are impossible in all situations, but more help can be given to the family by listening and explaining than by meeting the aggression with dismissive behaviour or counter-aggression. When explaining, however, it is important to remember that all information given should be based on the truth. It is better to say "I cannot be certain" in answer to queries about the child's condition than falsely to reassure the parents. Oakshot (1973) states that "fears of an ill child cannot be clearly visualised without allowing for the anxiety of the parents. In calming the parents and helping to relieve their anxiety the child will also be helped." If the parents have accompanied their child to hospital they may be in great distress, and, if they wish it, they should be encouraged to stay with their child. Alternatively, they should be offered somewhere to wait on their own and be kept informed of the child's progress at regular intervals. If possible a nurse should remain with them.

Police officers who have been called to the scene of an accident will often wait with the parents and be generally very supportive. Much information can be gained from the police and ambulance personnel who were present at the scene of the accident and full advantage should be taken of this additional source of information. Good relationships and liaison between the Accident and Emergency Department staff and the emergency services personnel are essential in these situations.

Specific Treatments in the Accident and Emergency Department
(where not mentioned elsewhere)

Unconscious Patients

The doctor is informed immediately that the child is expected or has arrived so that an examination can take place without delay. Maintenance of a clear airway is the first priority. An oral airway of the appropriate size can, if necessary, be inserted by the nurse on admission. Copious nasal and oropharyngeal secretions should be cleared regularly by suction. Clear nasal secretions should be tested for the presence of glucose to rule out the possibility of cerebrospinal fluid leakage. A nasogastric tube is passed by the doctor to empty the stomach and thus to prevent aspiration of gastric contents. The child should be placed in the semi-prone position if the possibility of cervical spine injury has been excluded. Oxygen is given as necessary if the child is cyanosed.

The focus of care then becomes one of careful observation. Pulse, respiration and blood pressure are taken and recorded. This is repeated at regular intervals (quarter-hourly until stable). A rise in intracranial pressure may be shown by a rise in the blood pressure, with slowing of the pulse and irregular breathing. Haemorrhage will cause a rapid pulse, with a low blood pressure and irregular respiration. Observation of pupil size and reaction is also made. Direct eye injuries will cause unequal pupil reaction and this should be considered, along with the possibility of raised intracranial pressure.

The time at which observations are made is noted so that improvement or deterioration can be easily monitored. Many hospitals have standard charts to make the recording of levels of consciousness less subjective, e.g. the Glasgow Coma Scale (Allan, 1986). To aid this, however, one nurse should be responsible for all recording during the child's stay in the department. If a skull fracture is suspected, an X-ray of the skull will be taken and consideration given to the advisability of obtaining radiographs of the cervical spine. The nurse should ensure that suction equipment and oxygen are available in the X-ray Department. Where possible, a portable radiographic examination performed in the resuscitation room is more satisfactory.

If a history is not available (e.g. if no-one accompanies the child) and trauma is not obvious, a cause of unconsciousness other than head injury, e.g. post-epileptic or diabetic coma, has to be considered. A drug or poison overdose may also be responsible. Parents should be asked about all drugs and poisons available to the child, not only the child's own drugs or the parent's but also those of grandparents or other family members to which the child has access. If poisoning is suspected, treatment should be given swiftly in liaison with the paediatrician and the poisons advice centre, and if the child is unconscious, it may be necessary to perform a gastric lavage – although this should be performed only by a doctor, with an anaesthetist present. The child should be intubated with a cuffed endotracheal tube to prevent the aspiration of stomach contents. (See Chapter 11 for the management of poisoning.)

A child who is or has been unconscious will be admitted to the ward. The nurse must remain with the unconscious child at all times. Suction equipment and oxygen should be available when the child is taken from the department to the ward for admission or to other departments for investigation. A portable suction unit and oxygen cylinder should be carried on the patient's trolley. Equipment for intubation and resuscitation and appropriate connections for oxygen cylinders should also be available, both on the trolley and in the departments to which a child is likely to be taken.

Fingertip Injuries

Trapped fingers and amputated fingertips are common accidents in children, usually occurring when a child traps his fingers in a door. Great distress and guilt are shown by the parents, who have often slammed the car or house door themselves. The child is also very distressed and frightened by the suddenness of events, his parent's reactions and often of the amount of blood in evidence. Injured fingertips usually bleed profusely. Amputated finger ends are not usually painful and older children when they have calmed down, often complain only of dull throbbing. Smaller children will become less distressed as their parents are reassured and calmed. As already described, the child can be distracted by toys and play. A sterile gauze dressing can be applied, with pressure until the bleeding stops. Parents can be reassured of the good results achieved in the regrowth of the finger, especially in children under 10 years of age. Photographs of healing and healed fingers are useful for this purpose.

Suturing of an avulsed fingertip is not necessary. Sterile adhesive strips, such as Steristrip or Ethistrip, are used to hold the cleansed and repositioned fingertip in place. A non-adherent dressing is then applied and held in place with a mitten bandage for small children and a fingertip bandage for older children. Parents should be advised to keep the dressing dry and in place until their return visit. This is not easy with active young children, so good bandaging is essential. Tape is not put completely around the wrist or finger because it will cause a constriction if swelling occurs. The dressing is usually changed in the Accident and Emergency Department after 24 hours to prevent it adhering to the wound. The parents should be told to return to the department with the child if the dressing gets wet or in 7–10 days to have it checked.

Amputated fingertips are dressed with Vaseline tulle, for example gauze Jelonet, and a well-padded bandage. A return visit in 7–10 days is necessary. Parents should be warned that the fingertip often looks unsightly when first seen. In two or three weeks, however, healing will be seen to be taking place. In the under-10s, in particular, the nail and finger-ends will regrow.

Lacerations

Bleeding is stopped by firm pressure on the wound with a sterile gauze pad, but if the laceration is caused by broken glass, pressure on the *edge* of the wound should be applied so that glass fragments do not penetrate further. When the bleeding has stopped, the wound can be inspected. Scalp lacerations and fingertip injuries all bleed profusely and often the extent of the wound cannot be seen until it is cleaned. If the laceration is over a tendon, movement of the limb and digit should be demonstrated, together with sensation, to check on possible nerve impairment. Colour should also be checked in case of impaired circulation. Regular observation and recording of these signs are then made until treatment is given.

Most children's lacerations can be closed with Steristrips or Ethistrips: these give a neater scar, do not act as a foreign body and save the trauma of sutures. Accurate application of the strips is essential for good results. The skin edges should be aligned carefully and adequate space left between the strips for air to circulate. Tincture of Benzoin applied to the skin around the laceration, except near the eyes or mouth, helps the strips to adhere. The wound is covered with a non-adherent dressing so that removal is easier. Facial wounds heal well when the strips are left exposed and generally even small children do not remove them when told firmly not to do so, especially if given the reasons why. The strips should be kept dry and left in position slightly longer than sutures.

Steristrips are not used when the wound is too large or if the area is unsuitable, for example over a joint or on the scalp. Suturing in small children may require a general anaesthetic, as they will not be co-operative if a local anaesthetic is used. When the laceration is over a joint, the limb is immobilised with a splint or a modified Robert Jones bandage. Knee sutures are inspected 48 hours after insertion to check for infection. Very dirty wounds, especially over the knee, are usually scrubbed. A general anaesthetic may be necessary for this. The joint should then be X-rayed.

Scalp lacerations can be closed successfully by using the child's hair knotted over the wound. The hair has to be of sufficient length and it helps the knots to hold if all the blood is not cleaned off the surrounding hair. The knot pulls the skin edges together and the clotted blood holds the knot in place. The knots are left in place for 7–10 days and then the hair strands of the knot are cut near to the scalp; the knots will then fall off with the scab. This method is less painful than suturing, and although it does pull the hair, it has the advantage of ease of application. No materials are needed other than the child's hair and nimble fingers. If knotting is impossible, the hair around the laceration should be shaved before suturing; sutures are removed after 5–7 days.

Tongue lacerations are not normally sutured and will heal very quickly, with no malformation, if left. Mouth washes should be given to the child after every meal to remove food particles from the wound. This is sometimes very difficult in young children and parents should be told to return if they are having problems. Some lip lacerations also do not require suturing. In any event, very small children will often chew on sutures around the mouth until they come out. If the lip is sutured, a topical local anaesthetic can be applied using a cotton wool swab prior to an injection of lignocaine.

Discharge from Hospital

When a child is discharged from the Accident and Emergency Department, written instructions together with verbal advice on any further care necessary should be given to his parents. Where possible, care should be continued by the community nursing team, especially if return to the Accident and Emergency Department would cause problems for the family.

Continuity of care from the hospital to the community services will be essential. A copy of the child's notes together with an account of the advice given or a comprehensive letter from the Accident and Emergency doctor should be forwarded to the GP. It is usual then for care to be continued by the health visitor, school nurse or community nurse. For this reason all information received from the hospital should be forwarded to the appropriate person. It is also helpful if, in addition to the usual written request for attendance, verbal liaison can take place between hospital and community staff. This will enable the primary health-care worker to have, in advance, an awareness of the child's needs and also gives her a chance to put any pertinent questions to the hospital staff. When the child is discharged it is important that his parents or guardian should understand that they can return to the department with the child should further treatment be needed or advice required.

Return Visit

How a child is treated on his first visit to hospital will influence his mood and behaviour on subsequent visits: unless very young, he will not forget the experience. The return visit is likely to be less traumatic, as injuries may have healed and the child will be prepared for the visit, but a caring, patient approach will still be necessary to elicit the best response from him. It will be less traumatic if children who are returning to the department can be seen and treated separately from children coming in as emergency admissions, perhaps with a separate waiting area and an appointment system.

As with emergency admissions, identification of the doctor and nurse attending the child is important. Where possible the child should be seen by the nurse who attended him initially; if there is an appointment system, it may be possible to arrange this. The doctor should signal the treatment prescribed and the nurse should sign the treatment record sheet when this has been given. The nurse should also report to the doctor any further information or observations on the child's condition or on the effects of treatment. Often parents will confide details to the nurse that they will omit to tell the doctor. Throughout the visit opportunities for play should be provided. Before the family leaves the department, accident prevention advice should be reinforced.

In Patient

If the child is to be admitted to hospital from the Accident and Emergency Department, all information gained and treatment given in the department should be relayed to the ward. The child's notes, observation charts, X-rays and other relevant material, such as drug containers or berries in accidental poisoning, should accompany the child to the ward, together with any information that might assist the ward staff in formulating the child's care plan.

The medical staff will already have communicated with each other when arranging admission and the senior Accident and Emergency and ward nurses should also communicate. All important information can be relayed verbally, but this must be backed up by the written information as soon as possible.

Ideally, the process of caring that commences in the Accident and Emergency Department should continue in the ward without any repetition of observations, treatment or in the gathering of personal and accident details. When time allows, such information, together with the objectives and outcome of care already given in the Accident and Emergency Department, should be entered into the nursing records. This will aid the process of continuity in the child's care.

Preparing the child and parents for admission is extremely important. The reasons for admission, procedures on the ward and details of any further treatment that may be given, including anaesthetics and operations, should be explained. General information about ward routine, visiting times, parent accommodation and facilities should also be given. Oakshot (1973) states that children's main anxieties are about separation from home, strange hospital procedures, anticipation of the anaesthetic and the operation itself. Explanation and reassurance on all aspects of the child's stay will help to prevent such anxiety.

A nurse, preferably the one who has been caring for the child in the Accident and Emergency Department, should accompany the child into the ward and give a verbal handover of information to the ward nurse.

Dealing with Death

Most professionals do not find this easy. Death is not a socially acceptable topic of conversation nor one with which people feel comfortable. In an emergency, death has not been expected and the parents are unprepared for it, everyone will be distressed. The parents should be treated with sympathy and given an opportunity to see and hold their child, in private if they wish. The child should be cleaned and dressed and any wounds should be covered, in order to help to make the experience less traumatic for his parents. It also helps if the child is placed in a less clinical area of the department while his parents see him. If the parents do not attend with the child, they should be allowed access to him in the mortuary or chapel of rest. A photograph taken of the child may help the parents at a later date, but this should not be thrust upon them unsolicited.

The documentation involved can wait until the following day, unless permission for a post-mortem examination is needed, because the parents will find it difficult to absorb information in their distressed state. Instructions on when to return to collect the information should be both given verbally to the parents and written down for them.

The health visitor should be informed of the death, so that she can offer support to the family and ensure that no appointments for routine treatments, such as immunisation, are sent to the dead child, which would only cause further distress to his parents.

Parents have commented that verbal expressions of grief by staff on the death of their child do not aid them as much as physical demonstrations of their sympathy. Comfort can be given by touching the person's hand or providing a shoulder to cry on.

Ethnic groups usually have extended families and strong support groups through their community or religion. As far as possible their customs concerning the child's body should be adhered to, but some procedures, such as post-mortem examination, cannot be disregarded. They should, however, be treated sympathetically, and as much leeway as is practical should be given. The nurse must be aware of ethnic customs and how these groups view death. The possibility of the dying child being a potential donor for a transplant programme should not be forgotten. This difficult matter is discussed in Chapter 4.

Medicolegal Problems

All notes, charts and diagrams made at the time of attendance may be used in future police or court proceedings. This should be borne in mind when any observations, recordings and treatment are undertaken. All observations should be recorded and documented in full with the date and time. Treatment should be given as prescribed and signed for after it has been carried out.

Accurate record-keeping is essential in case the information is required at a later date; memory is unreliable and not conducive to precise recall.

Children under the age of consent (16) should not be treated, except in exceptional circumstances, without the permission of their parents or guardian. This applies especially to invasive treatments such as injections and suturing.

References

Allan D (1986) The management of the head injured patient. *Nursing Times*, **82**(25): 36–39.

Hyson M C (1983) Going to the doctor: a developmental study of stress and coping. *Journal of Child Psychology and Psychiatry*, **24**(2): 247–259.

Richmond P W, Evans R C and Sibert J R (1987) Improving facilities in an accident department. *Archives of Diseases in Childhood*, **62**: 299–301.

Steering Group on Health Services Information, Korner Report (1982) *First Report to the Secretary of State* (Court Report). London: HMSO.

Chapter 4
Nursing Management of the Injured Child in the Ward
Donna Mead

When an injured child is admitted to hospital, the implications are either that the injuries sustained are serious enough to warrant treatment and care in hospital or that a period of careful observation is necessary, for example, following a head injury. Children are not always with their parents at the time of injury and in this event the child may be brought into hospital unaccompanied. When this occurs it is the responsibility of the nursing staff to ensure that the parents have been informed of the accident.

Whatever the circumstances, the typical picture on admission is one of a fretful and frightened child accompanied by anxious parents, whose anxiety is often made worse if they feel guilty or inadequate because their child has been involved in an accident.

It is usual then for the child and his family to have spent some time in the Accident and Emergency Department prior to transfer to the ward. When the child arrives in the ward, the first priority of the nursing staff will be to undertake those nursing actions that will enable him to recover from the physical aspects of his injuries. These actions include pain relief if necessary, as this is essential in promoting recovery. As these measures are discussed in the appropriate chapters, the purpose here is to outline the nursing actions necessary to assist the child and family to cope with and overcome the psychological and emotional trauma that results from an accident and to suggest a plan for accident prevention.

Immediate Care of the Injured Child

An initial assessment may be made in the Accident and Emergency Department and the information obtained given to the ward staff during the transfer. When this has not happened, this part of the assessment of the child should take place as soon as possible after his arrival in the ward.

The nurse should take into account the following factors when making the initial assessment of the child:

1. The child will not have been prepared for admission to hospital and thus any fears or misconceptions he may have about coming into hospital will be unresolved.
2. It is not uncommon for children to be warned about impending danger with the following proviso from parents: 'If you go out on to the road you'll have an accident and end up in hospital.' Where this is the case the hospital may be viewed as a place for punishment or the child may feel that his parents will be angered because their warning was ignored, or both.
3. The events surrounding the accident may be such that on admission to hospital the child remains very frightened.

Where levels of anxiety are high because of these factors the child may be either fractious and crying, and appear to be unco-operative, or quiet and withdrawn. The immediate goals in these circumstances will be to:

● gain the child's co-operation and trust,
● reduce anxiety to an acceptable level.

The nursing actions necessary to achieve these goals include:

1. Creating an environment that is calm and unhurried – one that is conducive to comforting and reassuring the child.
2. Ensuring that the child understands that someone will stay with him. Whenever appropriate, this person should be one or both of his parents. However, the extent of the injuries may be such that the parents may be apprehensive about holding their child. To the experienced nurse the intravenous infusion equipment presents little or no barrier to nursing the child, but to parents such equipment might constitute an insurmountable barrier to giving cuddles. As being cuddled by his parents is the action most likely to calm the child and reduce distress, it is important that the nurse should ensure that the parents are confident with their child. This is best achieved by the nurse demonstrating how these actions are possible and staying with the parents until they can handle their child with confidence.
3. Gaining the co-operation and trust of the child. Depending upon the child's age, this may be achieved by telling him about his injuries and why he is in hospital. There is a general consensus that children should be prepared to undergo procedures, painful or otherwise (Visintainer and Wolfer, 1975; Moss, 1981; Pinkerton, 1980). It is usually agreed that children need and are eager to know what is going to happen to them, that they need to be forewarned, that they expect honesty and that they will become very uncooperative if any part of the procedure is different from that which was explained to them. Such explanations should be geared to the child's stage of development and understanding. Perrin and Perrin (1983) noted that medical and nursing staff tend to underestimate the understanding of older children (11–15 years) and to overestimate that of younger children (5–11 years). It is important also to remember that children disregard the information they do not understand and become frustrated if "talked down"

to. What to tell the child and who should do the telling will depend on the nurse's assessments of the patient's need and desire to know and on his ability to comprehend. Rodin (1983) demonstrated the suitability of games and books as aids in preparing a child for painful procedures.

An initial assessment of the parents is made in the same way. When doing so the nurse should take into account the following factors:

1. The parents may be experiencing a range of emotions that include anxiety and might also involve guilt and reproach. When this is so the parents will typically be very tense and highly stressed.
2. Although the parents may already have been questioned at length while in the Accident and Emergency Department, the ward staff must also have specific details about the accident. However, it is important to ensure that the parents are not further distressed by what would appear to be constant questioning, because their being asked about the accident yet again may only have the effect of reinforcing what are often unfounded feelings of inadequacy or blame. This is particularly likely to be the case when parents feel that their negligence was responsible for the accident. If such feelings are allowed to develop as a result of constant questioning, the result will be a barrier to trust, co-operation and communication between the parents and nursing staff.
3. The converse might be the case and the parents may derive much comfort and relief, even at this stage, from talking about the accident and verbalising their fears.

The immediate goals at this stage will be to:

● gain the parents' co-operation and trust;
● alleviate anxiety or restore it to an acceptable level;
● preserve the existing relationship between parents and child by ensuring that it is not compromised by any feelings of inadequacy or guilt that the parents may have.

The nursing actions necessary to achieve these goals include:

1. Where possible, obtaining the necessary information relating to the accident itself from the Accident and Emergency staff.
2. When parents are obviously distressed about the accident, asking only those questions necessary to obtain information about their child's normal behaviour, for example, his sleeping pattern. For the parents this approach will demonstrate that the staff are not dwelling on the accident but rather are interested in the current needs of the child.
3. If the parents' needs are such that they must verbalise their fears and express their feelings of guilt, ensuring that appropriate facilities are made available for them to do this. Such facilities might include a room away from the child, where privacy can be ensured and interruptions avoided. A nurse should be available to take the time to listen to the parents' fears and anxieties.
4. Whatever the circumstances that caused the accident, it is advisable to

refrain at this stage from offering suggestions for avoiding a repetition of the accident or appearing to be judgmental in any way. Where the parents invite comment from the nursing staff, it might be better to inform them that over the next few days they may like to review the circumstances of the accident again, together with the nursing and medical staff, to see what can be learned from it. A positive approach of this nature will do much to preserve the parents' self-esteem.

5. Careful explanation of all procedures, as this will assist in alleviating parental anxiety. Such action demonstrates that the nursing staff intend to keep the parents informed and involved. Where feelings of guilt prevail, some parents may mistakenly think that because of their negligence the professionals have taken over the care of the child. This is not so and it is the responsibility of the nursing staff to promote a feeling of partnership between parents and staff.

6. Ensuring that the parents realise that they are welcome to stay with their child for as long as they would like. At the same time, the nurse should ensure that the parents' feelings of guilt in relation to the accident are not made worse by the fact that they have to return home to care for siblings. Where such a situation arises the nurse should reassure the parents that the child will be adequately cared for in their absence. Where the parents would be able to stay with their injured child if they could reorganise arrangements at home, e.g. care of pets or collecting siblings from school, the nurse should do anything she can to help, for example by providing the use of a telephone.

Such actions are necessary to restore the parents' confidence and to preserve their self-esteem, and are essential for the successful outcome of the subsequent programme of accident prevention.

It should be remembered that the extent to which the parents' anxiety can be alleviated will depend upon the nature of the injuries and what is known about their outcome. Where facial injuries or burns have occurred, for example, the parents will be worried about scarring. This is a legitimate worry: they will want to hear that there will be no scarring. However, it would be quite dishonest and destructive to any future relationship to reassure the parents by telling them what they want to hear if it is likely to be untrue. It is often very difficult to estimate how much scarring will result, and when the injuries are major it is often difficult initially to estimate whether or not impairment, disability or handicap will result. Even when surrounded by such uncertainty, the nurse should always give the parents an honest answer.

The Child's Ongoing Needs

As the child's physical condition becomes more stable and a relationship of trust and confidence is established, the focus of nursing care is on:

● minimising the psychological effects of the accident, if any exist;
● preventing a re-occurrence of such an accident.

The ward-based nursing staff are often thwarted in this task because when the injuries are minor, the child is ready for discharge by this time. Where such a situation exists it is important that the paediatric health visitor liaison is thoroughly briefed by the ward staff about the child, his parents and the accident, to ensure adequate follow up so that the effects of the accident on the family can be monitored, the family and home circumstances assessed and the appropriate programme of accident prevention instigated.

Where the nature of the injuries are such that the child is expected to stay in hospital for some time, it is the responsibility of the ward-based staff to liaise with health visitor colleagues to consider how such care can be best achieved. This will be based on:

1. *an assessment of the child's understanding of the accident.*   Depending on the child's age, this may be arrived at through play or open discussion. If, following discussion with medical colleagues, it is felt that re-enactment of the events might lead to a better understanding of how the accident occurred, this approach should be used to aid the assessment.

2. *an assessment of the psychological effects of the accident on the child.*   Before such an assessment can be made the nurse will need to know about the child's usual routines and habits, for instance his usual patterns of sleeping, eating and playing. She can then gauge the extent of the psychological effects of the accident by comparing his present behaviour with his behaviour before the accident.

The nursing actions necessary to minimise the effects of the accident include:

1. Observing carefully any changes in behaviour. All children regress when admitted to hospital, owing to insecurity and fear of the new environment, and it is important to remember that some changes in the child's behaviour pattern may be attributable to the effects of hospitalisation *per se*. It is essential, therefore, that the nurse is able to discriminate between the two. Regression may be manifested by thumb-sucking or by soiling or bed-wetting in a child who has previously been dry at night. The child may also become withdrawn or prone to aggressive outbursts and constantly demand attention. Observations, together with an assessment of the child's under-standing of the accident, enable the nurse to determine the extent to which the accident has affected the child psychologically.

2. Creating an environment in which the child is able to talk about his fears. In so doing the use of play, for example drawing, playing with dolls, teddies or Action Man, or merely observing the child at play with other children, is advocated. Often the child's fears are unfounded or have become distorted as a result of his imagination. It can be seen, therefore, that it is important to discover the nature of the child's fears, so that any misunderstandings can be cleared up.

3. Restoring the child's confidence so that he may become involved in similar situations without fearing another accident. This could involve an education programme appropriate to the child's level of understanding and knowledge of the accident. It is important to note that it is the responsibility of adults to create a safe environment for children. Educating the child must in no way

be seen as relinquishing this responsibility. However, it can be appreciated that if the child feels that he knows how to ensure that he is not involved in a similar accident, this will do much to restore his confidence. Also, the child may be of an age where safety consciousness is apparent, in which case the nursing staff should take advantage of this situation to foster such awareness.

4. Minimising the effects of boredom if a long period in hospital is necessary. This may be achieved by planning a programme of play that is appropriate to the child's stage of development while also taking into account the limitations resulting from the injuries incurred. (See Chapter 9 for suggestions of suitable play for a child with one or more limbs immobilised.)

5. Minimising the effects of separation from family and friends. Wolff (1969) describes a study by Schaeffer that showed the reaction of children from different age groups to separation from their family. The main aspects of separation and some suggestions for minimising the effects are described.

(a) *Babies under 7 months of age*
    The main problems in this age group are concerned with sensory deprivation on the part of the child. The parents and family will be the ones experiencing feelings of loss, guilt and other emotional problems resulting from being separated from the baby. For the baby, problems can be reduced by:

    • providing interesting toys at eye level;
    • adults talking and playing with the baby whenever they pass the cot or undertake procedures;
    • social approaches from older children on the ward who are up and about.

    Frequent visits by the family and their involvement in every aspect of the care of the baby will help both the baby and the family.

(b) *Babies 7–18 months old*
    The baby will initially show emotional reactions to being separated from his parents. He will cry a lot and 'talk' very little. When his parents do visit he will probably cling to them and react when they leave, making it very much more upsetting for them. After a few days, however, he will start to get used to his surroundings and gradually react less to the arrival and departure of his parents. However, it is essential that what appears to be settling in is not mistaken for detachment. There may also be problems when the baby returns home. He may show symptoms of 'over-dependence' on his parents, including clinging, wanting to be fed when he could previously feed himself and not wanting to be left alone. These usually last for about two weeks.

(c) *Todders 18 months to 4 years old*
    This age group does not readily accept a substitute for parents. Prugh (1953) showed that children of this age are disturbed while in hospital and can have behavioural disorders on discharge, no matter how much attention they received from nurses and other staff except when their mother is admitted with them to be in constant attendance.

(d) *Children 4 years of age and older*

Prugh also observed the behaviour of this age group. These children seem to be able to accept strangers more readily as parent substitutes after an initial period of getting to know them, but exhibit fewer long-term emotional problems if the number of strangers is limited to only those necessary to provide continuity.

Where possible, therefore, a primary nurse should be the sole person responsible for planning and supervising the care of a particular child throughout his stay in hospital. The best people to cater for the basic daily needs of these children are, of course, usually their parents. By promoting and encouraging a family-centred approach to care, the effects of separation can usually be minimised.

(e) *Adolescents*

The main problems with children of this age group are related to lack of privacy and lack of contact with peers at a time in their lives when both these aspects are becoming important to them. Some paediatric hospitals are developing adolescent wards, where these children can be nursed together and attention can be paid to their special needs. Where such facilities are not available the important aspects of care include:

- grouping similarly aged children together in bays or at one end of an open ward;
- using side rooms whenever possible to allow privacy;
- allowing any reasonable posters, photographs, magazines, etc. that the child wants around his bed;
- allowing certain freedoms from inappropriate hospital routines, e.g. allowing tea or coffee instead of fruit squashes and milk;
- letting them use their own sheets and bed coverings (Most children now have duvets, not blankets, and may prefer them.);
- letting them dress in their own clothes where possible. Even if the child has his legs immobilised by traction and cannot wear trousers, he can still wear his own T-shirt or shirt. Shorts or a skirt can be adapted by undoing the side seams and replacing them with velcro or ties. They can be worn easily with POP casts or traction. T-shirt dresses and other tops can be adapted in the same way if the child has a POP cast or traction to the arm.

The Parents Ongoing Needs

It is at this time, when the child is recovering and the parents and nursing and medical staff have established a relationship of trust and co-operation, that attention will be given to preparing the parents for the child's discharge, and that the nursing staff will need to work closely with community colleagues. Such preparation begins with an assessment of the factors that may place members of the family at high risk of further accidents (Table 4.1).

Table 4.1 High-risk factors involved in a family's susceptibility to accidents

Risk Factor	Example
Family size	Several children with little support from husband
Stress	Mother taking antidepressants/tranquillisers
Lack of awareness on the part of parents	Allowing very young children to go to school unaccompanied
Ergonomic factors	Glass doors that are not fitted with safety-glass in a home with small children
Economic factors	Insufficient funds for fire guards, safety-glass, etc.

Risks based on the factors listed in Table 4.1 are identified and analysed to see which of them can be eliminated, and the parents' ability to understand the nature of and participate in an education for prevention programme is assessed. As a result of this assessment the goals of care will be focused on:

● accident prevention, such that by the time of discharge the parents will feel equipped to prevent a recurrence of the accident;
● eliminating the risk factors that have been identified.

The nursing actions necessary to achieve these goals include:

1. Ensuring that the parents understand the sequence of events that led up to the accident. There is some evidence that one-to-one teaching in families who are at risk from accidents is beneficial (Colver et al, 1982). The period during which the child is recovering in hospital is a suitable time for such teaching because the nursing staff have an opportunity to design a teaching programme to cater for the family's needs.

   Gaffin (1981) suggests that three interlinked factors are involved in the examination of an accident: the child, the agent involved and the environment (physical or social). Figure 4.1 shows how these factors can be represented diagrammatically for teaching purposes.

   This approach is a useful one because it allows parents to consider the interlinking factors in the accident, thereby facilitating significant learning, and is more effective than simply 'telling' the parents how the accident happened.

2. Enabling the parents to plan an accident prevention programme for their family. This is possible only when an understanding of the interlinking factors involved in the accident has been achieved. Such a plan would need to focus on accidents in general as well as on the particular accident in which the child was involved.

3. Ensuring that the parents are aware of the kind of support available from different agencies, where this is appropriate, e.g. the DSS when there is financial hardship, so that safety gates or fireguards may be provided, or the Home Safety Officer for safety advice.

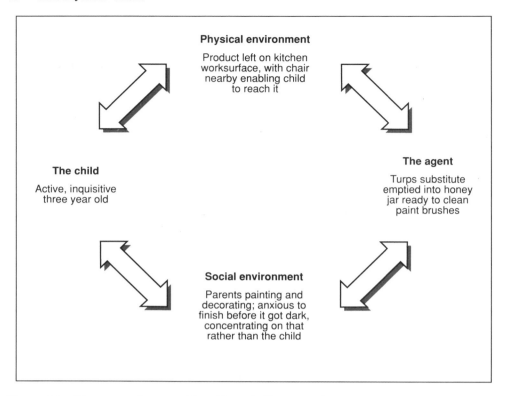

Figure 4.1   The aspects in an accident (from Gaffin, 1981. Reproduced by kind permission of Medical Education [International] Ltd)

The Nurse's Role in Caring for a Child who is Disabled or Handicapped as a Result of an Accident

It is difficult to define the term 'handicap'. It may be measured in terms of a functional loss, such as that which results from the loss of a limb or finger. It may also be measured in terms of a sensory handicap, such as partial or complete loss of sight and hearing. Jackson (1981) noted that the problem of definition is compounded by the lack of any studies that provide objective data relating to the measurement of handicap. 'Accident plus child equals what in terms of disability?' is the question he poses.

If the long-term effect of accidents is examined from a broader perspective than that of purely locomotor handicap, the following picture emerges:

- 1.5 per cent of all children admitted to hospital with head injuries do have residual neurological handicap, i.e. about 2000 children per year (Jamison and Kaye, 1974).
- There are more eyes lost in the first decade of life than at any other time. Crombie (1981) argues that in up to 30 per cent of cases perforating injuries lead to the loss of an eye, which in absolute terms means that in the UK approximately 350 children's eyes are lost following injury each year. The

impairment that occurs as a result, for example loss of depth perception, lasts for life.

- Ten in every 1000 children aged less than 14 years (1 per cent of children each year) are at risk of becoming disabled from accidents (Harker, 1981, based on epidemiological studies in Liverpool).
- Following a fatal drowning accident, 24 per cent of parents in a study of drowning in Brisbane (Nixon and Pearn, 1977) separated.

How do the implications of these findings affect the nurse caring for the injured child in the ward? This question can best be answered by considering the children who fall into the following categories:

1. Those for whom it is obvious at the time of injury that handicap or disability will result.
2. Those for whom the physical/psychological/intellectual effects are not apparent at the time of injury.
3. Those who return to hospital regularly for treatment following an accident, for example as a result of burns.

A nurse working in a paediatric setting is likely to meet one or more children from each of these categories at some point during her practice and will, therefore, need to develop strategies for dealing with such children and their families.

When the parents realise that their child will be disabled as a result of the injuries incurred in the accident they may be overwhelmed with feelings of guilt; as a result they often become over-protective and this is sometimes manifest as over-indulging the child. The consequences of this sort of approach vary but may result in:

1. a child who is prevented from gaining full independence;
2. a child who is labelled 'spoiled' and who becomes selfish;
3. a child who is disliked by his siblings as a result of what they interpret as his receiving preferential treatment from the parents.

The end result is an increase of tension and stress within the family, with the ensuing high risk of marital breakdown.

It is the responsibility of the nurse who cares for the child at the time of the injury tactfully to point out these consequences to the parents. Experience suggests, for example, that it is not unusual for the child's cubicle to resemble the toy department of a large store within two or three days of the accident. Where this has happened the nurse can use the fact to demonstrate to the parents that they are already well on the way to the very undesirable outcome of a 'spoiled' child.

It is often very difficult for parents who are already devastated by the knowledge that their child will be disabled to accept this sort of information, but there are several strategies that the nurse may adopt:

1. Demonstrating to the parents the benefits to be gained from a firm but loving approach.
2. Ensuring that siblings are not neglected. The parents should spend time

with siblings as well as with the injured child. Although brothers and sisters are welcome in the paediatric ward, it is important that a sense of normality should be preserved for them also. This may best be achieved by parents spending some time at home with them as well as as much time as possible in the hospital with the injured child.

3. Encouraging parents who are currently caring for a child who is disabled as a result of an accident and who have coped with the necessary adjustments to be supportive of the parents of a recently disabled child. A list of the names and addresses of parents who are prepared to help in this way could be kept by the ward staff so that meetings can be arranged when it is felt that such action would benefit parents who are finding it difficult to adjust to their new circumstances.

If the nature of the injuries is such that the long-term effects are not apparent at the time of the accident, e.g. post-traumatic epilepsy, the parents will obviously not have received support of the sort outlined above. Such support becomes necessary as the effects become apparent and may be given by ward-based staff if admission to hospital is necessary or by the primary health-care team, who may involve colleagues from other disciplines, e.g. the physiotherapist or social worker.

The child who is admitted to hospital regularly as a result of his injuries faces the following problems:

● Interrupted schooling.
● Repeated separation from family and friends.
● Difficulty in developing his physical, social and psychological potential as fully as possible.
● Refusal to co-operate when frequent hospital admissions are necessary.
● Altered body image.

The nursing actions necessary to overcome these problems are discussed under the relevant headings, as follows:

Interrupted Schooling

When it is inevitable that frequent hospital admissions will interrupt the child's schooling the hospital school teacher should liaise with the child's own school to maintain continuity and to prevent the child from falling behind. This is particularly important in older children who are studying for major examinations, and if absence is prolonged individual tuition at home or in hospital can be arranged through the Social Services Department.

If no teachers are available, nurses can promote an educational environment by creating a regular routine for the day where so far as possible, school hours are kept for educational activities and play is allowed after school hours. Careful use of video, television and educational audio-cassettes is a good idea. Work books and reading lists may be available from the local educational board, or the child's own teachers may be able to provide appropriate material and learning programmes, which parents can help to plan.

Repeated Separation

This is a particularly difficult problem to overcome, especially if the child's injuries are such that specialist treatment is required at a regional centre some distance from home and if his mother cannot therefore be resident in the hospital. Depending on the child's age, contact with family and friends may be maintained by letter and/or taped messages; photographs of family members, pets, friends (e.g. a class photograph, Brownie or Cub Pack), can be displayed as the child wishes. Every effort should be made to facilitate visits from family and friends, and for the parents to stay and be involved in their child's care.

Primary Nursing is recommended as one way of ameliorating the effects of repeated separation because it limits the number of contacts the child has with different health professionals and facilitates bonding with the primary and associate nurses.

Developmental Difficulties

The child may be faced with the problem of limited physical development as a result of the accident and if he is subjected to teasing from friends, his psychosocial development might also be impaired. Nursing staff and parents alike will need much patience and understanding in order to help the child overcome problems of this sort.

It is important to remember that it is through play that children develop many physical, social and psychological skills. Where necessary, play may have to be modified and toys carefully chosen, so that the child continues to develop to his full potential through this medium. Assistance from a play therapist may be useful in this regard. It is also important that the child's environment in hospital or at home is such that he is able to develop with confidence and self-esteem.

Refusal to Co-operate

The nurse should be aware that the basis for such behaviour is often frustration or anger at repeated interruptions to normal routine or life-style. It is important always to be honest with a child, as children of all ages can generally cope better with the truth than with their own, vivid imagination or fear of the unknown. All explanations must be geared to the child's level of understanding. If ward nursing staff are not honest with a child, he may lose trust in them.

Altered Body Image

How this will affect the child will depend upon the extent of his injuries. These may range from a small scar to the loss of an eye, a shortened limb or extensive scarring from burns, all of which will have some effect on the child's perception of himself. As he grows it is inevitable that he will become more aware of his altered body image. Adolescence may be a particularly difficult time, as the young adult's body image will be detrimentally affected by any abnormality, no matter how slight. Early recognition of potential problems for this age group is important so that treatment and counselling can be provided, both for the adolescent himself and for his family. Where the adolescent has to accept physical limitations as a result of his injuries it may be possible to encourage him to develop other talents so that his self-esteem is preserved.

An important aspect of the nurse's role in caring for the child who is disabled or handicapped as a result of an accident is to ensure that the parents are aware of the support and facilities that are available and, where necessary, to put them in touch with the appropriate agency. Practical help is available from:

1. The National Health Service,   Consultant Community Physician
   including hospital   Members of the District Handicap Team
   and community services   Occupational Therapist
                            Physiotherapist
                            Psychologist
                            Speech therapist
2. The education department (local education authority)
3. Social Services Department

It is usually the social worker who co-ordinates all these services for the family. The contribution of voluntary agencies and self-help groups is also very helpful and the ward nursing staff should be able to put parents in touch with organisations of this nature. A list of useful addresses is given at the end of this chapter.

When a Child Dies as a Result of an Accident

There are many excellent texts that deal with the care of the child who dies, either suddenly or following a protracted illness at home or in hospital (see the list of recommended reading at the end of this chapter). When a child dies as result of an accident, this has a profound and lasting effect on his family. Parents may experience not only a sense of failure but also one of overwhelming guilt. It is the nature of these effects that will be dealt with here.

When death is inevitable the nurse must ensure that she does nothing either by her actions or in what she says that will give the parents something with which to reproach themselves later. As part of the grieving process the parents may relive the final days over and over again, examining in minute detail every conversation held with nursing and medical staff. Unfortunately, in an effort to be reassuring the nurse may be sowing the seeds for the parents' feelings of added guilt. For example, the nurse who says 'You must not blame yourself, you cannot be expected to be everywhere' may not have taken into account that this thought may not yet have occurred to the parents, and if considered carefully it can be seen that this is a 'stock phrase' and forms no part of an individualised approach to care.

If the injuries are horrific, it is important for the parents to understand that their child is not suffering. As well as ensuring that adequate analgesia is given, a calm, peaceful and unhurried environment is necessary.

The parents should be allowed as much involvement in care as they wish up to and after the time of his death. It is important that facilities that ensure privacy for the family are made available.

A child who dies as a result of an accident may well be a suitable donor for organs such as kidneys, and it is the responsibility of the medical staff to approach the parents to request permission for their removal. Experience suggests that, when circumstances permit, it is better to obtain the parents' decision before death has occurred. In any event, the situation is stressful for everyone involved and the role of the nurse in this instance is to support the parents and medical staff where possible. Inevitably the parents will later have many questions that they did not ask at the time of the request, and it is often to the nursing staff that these questions will be addressed. It is important that the nurse should endorse the comments already made by the doctors so that the facts remain clear, but this will be possible only if a member of the nursing staff was present at the earlier meeting and has communicated the outcome to her colleagues.

The nurse should support the parents by being available to listen to them, if required, when they discuss the issues and by ensuring privacy in a quiet room so that they will feel able to cry, embrace or express whatever emotions they wish in arriving at their decision.

The parents will also be faced with the fact that a post-mortem examination will be required by the coroner to determine the cause of death, and for many parents this prospect is an additional cause of much anguish.

It is important to remember that siblings are particularly vulnerable when a brother or sister dies, especially if the parents have been so involved with the dying child that they have had little or no time for others. Liddell (1981) has found that siblings who are given no help in understanding what is happening or in expressing anxieties may react by exhibiting behaviour disturbances that may eventually manifest as school phobia, regression or fear of illness. It is important, therefore, that siblings should remain part of the family circle and be kept informed of what is happening at a level appropriate to their understanding.

There are organisations, local and national, that provide support for bereaved parents and a list of local groups should be kept in every paediatric ward. The Compassionate Friends (for bereaved parents) is a national organisation: its address is

The Compassionate Friends
(for bereaved parents)
25 Kingsdown Parade
Bristol BS6 5UE

Other useful addresses are:

Dial UK
National Association of Disablement Information
Dial House
117 High Street
Clay Cross
Chesterfield
Derbyshire S45 9D2

Headway
National Head Injuries Association
200 Mansfield Road
Nottingham N61 3HX

Headway publications include:

Head Injuries and Epilepsy
Accident and Emergency Head Injuries: Advice for Relatives.

References

Colver A F, Hutchison P J and Judson E C (1982) Promoting children's home safety. *British Medical Journal*, **285**: 1177–1180.

Crombie A L (1981) *The Long Term Consequences of Accidents to Children.* In: Occasional Paper No. 4, London: The Child Accident Prevention Trust.

Gaffin J (1981) Accidents in the home, *Nursing*, (1st Series) **23**: 992–994.

Jackson H (1981) Disability and accidents: the unsolved equation in disability. In: *The Long Term Consequences of Accidents to Children*, ed. Crombie A L. Occasional Paper No. 4, London: The Child Accident Prevention Trust.

Jamison D L and Kaye H H (1974) Accidental head injury in childhood. *Archives of Diseases in Childhood*: **49**: 376–381.

Harker P (1981) Disability and accidents. In: *The Long Term Consequences of Accidents to Children*, ed. Crombie A L. Occasional Paper No. 4, London: The Child Accident Prevention Trust.

Liddell G (1981) Death of a child. *Nursing*, (1st Series) **34**: 1496–1497.

Moss J R (1981) Helping young children to cope with the physical examination. *Paediatric Nursing*, **7**: 17–20.

Nixon J and Pearn J H (1977) Emotional sequelae of parents and sibs, following drowning or near drowning of a child. *Journal of Psychology*, **11**: 265–268.

Perrin E and Perrin J (1983) Clinicians assessments of children's understanding of illness. *American Journal of Diseases in Childhood*, **137**(9): 874–878.

Pinkerton P (1980) Preparing children for surgery. *On Call*, 5th June: 8–9.

Prugh D (1953) A study of the emotional reactions of children and families to hospitalisation and illness. *American Journal of Orthopsychiatry*, **23**: 70.

Rodin J (1983) *Will This Hurt?* London: Royal College of Nursing.

Visintainer M A and Wolfer J A (1975) Psychological preparation for surgical paediatric patients: the effect on children's and parents' stress responses and adjustment. *Paediatrics*, **56**: 187–202.

Wolff S (1969) *Children Under Stress.* London: Trend and Co.

Recommended Reading

Bluebond-Langner M (1978) *The Private Worlds of Dying Children.* Princeton: Princeton University Press.

Keirs J A. *Change of Rhythm: The Consequences of a Road Accident.* Published by Jackie Kiers, 4 Edith Road, Oxford, OX1 4QA.

Kubler Ross E (1983) *On Children and Death.* New York: Macmillan. *Aspects of Sick Children's Nursing: A Learning Package*, Sections 56 and 57 (1982) Milton Keynes: General Nursing Council for England and Wales.

Chapter 5
Specific Accident Situations

J R Sibert   Donna Mead

Road Traffic Accidents

More children die from road traffic accidents (RTAs) than from any other accidental cause. This clearly presents a major challenge in prevention and treatment to all those who work in the field. Four-hundred-and-seven children died and 8620 were seriously injured in RTAs in 1986. Of those children who died, 266 were pedestrians and 33 were pedal cyclists. The figures of casualties from RTAs are almost certainly an underestimate, as they are based on police notifications and not on hospital statistics.

Pedestrian Road Traffic Accidents

Pedestrian road traffic accidents are particularly common in poorer areas and in children from socially deprived families. This has been shown in national death statistics and recently in a study from Sheffield (Sunderland, 1984): the fatality rate was universally related to the prosperity of the area. Psychosocial stress is also an important factor in road traffic accidents, as was shown by Backett and Johnson (1959). Indeed, it is probably the subtle interaction of a poor environment with stress that is involved in many accidents. It is easy to see how a mother with three children under five, living in a house with a door opening on to a road with heavy traffic, could easily have her attention diverted, so that one of them could run into the road and be injured.

The number of pedestrian road traffic accidents reaches a marked peak in children between five and seven years, with boys involved twice as often as girls (Routledge et al, 1974). This is the age when children first go to school, but have not yet learned the dangers of traffic and how to deal with it. Psychologists studying RTAs have constantly found that parents considerably overestimate the ability of children under eight to judge the speed and danger of cars adequately. As well as teaching children through programmes such as the Green Cross Code, parents also need educating so that they do not overestimate the ability of their children, providing supervision in traffic and if necessary accompanying the child to school.

The most effective way of preventing RTAs is by modification of the environment. This can be done by redesigning residential areas to give priority to pedestrians and to separate them from traffic. This has been accomplished in Sweden (Sandel, 1975). Such separation is more difficult to achieve in older, inner-city areas, where most accidents occur and many at-risk children live. There are a number of solutions that could be used together or singly, including pedestrian-only streets, streets with access only, and speed-reducing bumps ('sleeping policemen'). The provision of play areas will reduce the number of children playing in dangerous streets. Much of this is the responsibility of the local council, and where such changes in design are necessary, nurses should be active in informing council members of this need.

Passenger Accidents

Before legislation compelling the use of seat belts in the front seats of cars was introduced in 1983, children were injured and killed when travelling as passengers in both the front and rear seats. The majority of children probably now travel in the back seats, and, indeed, more children are killed and injured when travelling in the rear of cars than in the front. In a 1978 study by the Transport and Road Research Laboratory of child casualties in car accidents, 25 per cent of children dying in car accidents had been sitting in the front seat and the remaining 75 per cent in the rear.

In 1985 69 of the 457 children who died on the road died as car passengers. The protection of children in cars from serious injury and death must therefore be an important part of any child safety programme, whether on a national, local or individual level. A major part of such protection of children is the development of child restraint systems and seat belts. Avery (1980) stated that up to 1000 serious injuries to children could be prevented each year by the use of proper restraint systems.

Much of the research on seat belts has been on adult car passengers. There is good evidence that seat belts are effective in preventing death and serious injury. However, educational campaigns to persuade people to wear them have generally been unsuccessful. Since 1983, when legislation was introduced compelling the wearing of seat belts in front seats of vehicles, serious injuries have fallen by as much as 20 per cent. There is good evidence also that children's restraints prevent injury and death. The Transport and Road Research Laboratory found that, over a two-year period, no child died when in such a restraint, whereas 264 non-restrained child passengers were killed during this time. Scherz (1976) found that in the State of Washington, USA, serious injuries and deaths were much less common in restrained than unrestrained children, especially in younger age groups. Child restraints also had an unexpected bonus in that they improved children's behaviour, thus probably improving the parent's driving standards (Christopherson, 1977). Avery (1980) states that the single most effective action that a driver of a car can take to reduce the chances of injury during an accident (other than avoiding the accident in the first place) is to place the child in a restraint suitable for the child's age. It is argued that if this were routinely carried out for all children it is possible that as many as 50 to 70 children could avoid death and 1000 avoid serious injury in motor cars each year in the UK.

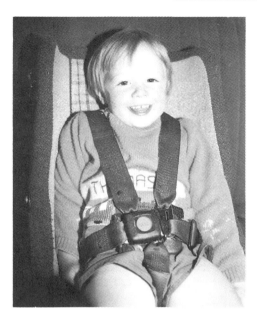

Figure 5.1   Child car seat (Reproduced by
kind permission of *Nursing Standard*)

The most suitable restraint very much depends upon the age of the child. For babies the safest way used to be the carry-cot restraint. These are no longer recommended because the cot rather than the baby itself is restrained. Recently a number of baby carriers for babies less than 10 kg (22 lb) in weight have been developed. These are portable seats that may be fixed to the car with an adult safety belt, these have proved to be convenient and safe in use and do restrain the baby. Their wider use can be encouraged by loan schemes.

Children weighing between 10 and 18 kg (22–40 lb) should ride in a child car seat (Figure 5.1), which can either be fixed directly to the car by two- or four-point anchorage or fitted with adult seat belts, the latter design being particularly convenient.

For children from 18–36 kg (40–80 lb) adult seat belts should be used with a booster cushion. These are as safe as child harnesses. Recent legislation covering cars fitted with rear seat belts requires children carried in such vehicles to be restrained by approved safety seats or belts.

British Standards for Child Restraint Systems
Baby carriers: BS AU202
Carry-cot restraints: BS AU186
Child car seats (two- or four-point anchorage): BS 3254 or ECE reg 44
Child car seats (for adult seat belts): BS 3254 or ECE reg 44
Booster cushions: BS AU185 or ECE reg 44
Child harnesses: BS 3254

Bicycle Injuries

Bicycles play an important part in the life of most children, particularly boys between three and 12 years of age. Injuries on bicycles cause about 5 per cent of all childhood accidents presenting to hospital, and they also cause a significant number of serious injuries and death. There is a marked increase in the incidence of bicycle accidents in summer and early autumn: from April to September hospital attendances are about five times those for October to May.

Boys outnumber girls by a factor of three in having bicycle injuries, and these accidents reach their peak at eight years of age. Of particular concern are head injuries; one in 600 boys between eight and 12 years old has a serious enough head injury to be admitted to hospital (under present criteria for head injury) per year. Put another way, one in 100 boys has a significant head injury while riding a bicycle during his childhood. Illingworth (1985) categorised the cause of 300 bicycle accidents as:

- Falling off after striking an object on the road.
- Hitting a bump in the road or a drain hole.
- Collision with lamp-posts or other fixed objects.
- Riding into the kerb.
- Slipping off the edge of the kerb.
- Riding into a parked car.
- Collision with or being hit by a moving car.
- Skidding – mostly on gravel.
- Falling after slipping off a pedal, seat or handlebar.
- Falling while changing gear.
- Objects being caught in spokes, pedals or chain.
- Unfamiliarity with the bicycle.
- Riding a bicycle that is too big.
- Riding two to a bicycle, or other pranks (Figure 5.2).

There are factors in bicycle design that are vital to safety. For instance, the 'high-rise' bicycle, which was introduced into Britain in the late 1960s and early 1970s, had features that made it more dangerous than standard models. These caused the centre of gravity to lie behind the back wheel when the rider was mounted, making the machine unstable, and the gear stick was placed in a way that caused severe genital injuries. Improvements in design have now meant that this model has been superceded.

More recently the widespread popularity of the BMX bicycle has caused concern, not so much because of any intrinsic dangerous design factor but because of the whole ethos of the bicycle, encouraging dangerous behaviour.

The question that remains unanswered is how to promote safety awareness in the cycle rider. Illingworth (1985) notes that many factors such as the child's personality and play behaviour, including racing and showing off, cannot and should not be altered. It would also be very difficult to prevent objects lying on the road and irregularities in the road surface. The prevention or reduction of severity of bicycle injuries may involve education and environmental change. Children under the age of nine should not be allowed in traffic, and at this age they should become involved in ROSPA's National Cycling Proficiency Scheme.

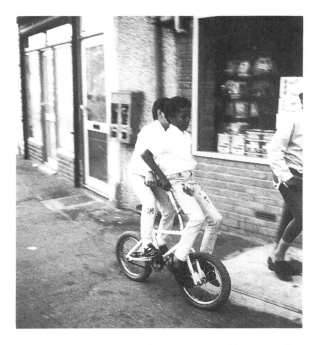

Figure 5.2   Bicycle pranks – many accidents causing
head injury result from this type of behaviour

In addition, more schools should be encouraged to adopt the Cycle Way road safety education package. Cycling proficiency courses should also include proper maintenance of chain, gears and brakes. However, no matter how effective such training becomes, children will always be found riding round residential streets for fun. It is thus essential that drivers anticipate any antics and themselves exhibit safe behaviour in these areas.

Parents should be encouraged to give thought to the type of bicycle they buy for their child or allow him to ride, as well as to protective clothing and helmets. BMX clubs ensure that protective clothing is worn, but Illingworth (1985) found that only two of the 300 children studied had ridden BMX bicycles and had worn protective clothing. Head protectors and helmets have been suggested as a way of reducing the severity of bicycle injuries, but at present, this type of protection is not easily available and is expensive. A first step in its more widespread use would be to ensure that helmets are cheap and easy to buy, and a publicity campaign is needed to encourage their use. A British Standard will soon be available in this area.

The promotion of special cycle tracks keeping children on bicycles away from traffic has improved the safety outlook, allowing them to ride quite long distances away from cars and other vehicles. Their provision must be included in any environmental safety scheme for an area.

Dog Bites

One in every hundred children presents to the Accident and Emergency Department each year with a dog bite. The majority of injuries are minor, but severe lacerations, particularly facial lacerations, do occur. There are a few deaths, mainly from children attacked by guard dogs.

In a study in the USA (Lauer et al, 1982) German Shepherd dogs (Alsatians) were the commonest breed of dog involved in dog bites to children. In the USA and the UK, many of the accidents occur in the home, or with dogs well known to the children, but a significant number of children are bitten whilst in public places, particularly play areas.

Dog bite cases are usually given tetanus prophylaxis, but routine antibiotics are not usually needed. In other countries, particularly in India, the danger of rabies is ever-present. Rabies has now reached the north coast of France and is only kept out of the UK by stringent quarantine and immigration regulations.

The health visitor has an important role in informing parents of the dangers of dogs, not only with respect to injuries, but also regarding toxocara infestation. Some areas have byelaws insisting that dogs are kept on the lead in parks and play areas.

Falls

Falls cause a significant number of deaths in childhood and are also the commonest cause of injury in children presenting to the Accident and Emergency Department (Sibert et al, 1981).

Falls, of course, have a varied aetiology and may be on one level, such as falling on the pavement or in the school playground. Many such falls occur as a result of unruly or poor behaviour. Better supervision of play may be the only way to prevent these injuries.

Falls can also be from one level to another, for instance from a tree while climbing, from windows or down the stairs. Little can be done to prevent falls from trees, but design factors can help prevent window and stair falls. Poor window catches cause a number of accidents, particularly in high-rise flats. The introduction of safety catches or window guards will reduce this sort of accident. Indeed, in New York City a programme providing free window guards (the 'Children Can't Fly' Programme – Spiegel and Linderman, 1977) has been successful in preventing window falls in a poor area of the city.

Falls down the stairs are particularly prevalent in toddlers and much can be done to prevent them by improving stair design. Open stairs with wide gaps between ballustrades may be aesthetically pleasing but are dangerous for young children. Stair gates may be valuable, especially for the busy mother in a poorly designed property. Their use can be encouraged by the health visitor. For those receiving Supplementary Benefit a Department of Social Security grant may be available for such gates, but it does not always cover the cost of two gates, which are recommended to guard both the head and the foot of the stairs.

The Child Accident Prevention Trust and the Royal Institute of British Architects, in order to encourage safer design for children in new houses, have published *Child Safety and Housing* (Page, 1985), which includes practical design guidelines for commissioning agencies, architects, designers and builders. Also outlined in this publication are guidelines for stairway design.

Injuries from Glass

Falls through glass may cause severe lacerations to hands, wrists, arms and occasionally the face. Severe damage may result from injury to arteries, nerves and tendons, and internal injuries may also be found, sometimes with the bowel protruding from the abdominal wall. It is estimated that there were 11,000 presentations to Accident and Emergency Departments from glass injuries in 1983 in the UK. There are also a few deaths each year, usually from uncontrolled arterial bleeding, and cases of scarring and permanent disability from nerve damage.

The child is usually injured by glass in doors or by low-level glazing. A typical story would be a child falling down the stairs into a glass door. The sharp jagged parts of the glass may cause severe lacerations to all parts of the body, particularly the upper limbs (Figure 5.3). First aid to sites of severe bleeding from glass injuries is best done by pressure on the wound, using a pad after the glass has been removed. In some cases quite extensive surgery is needed to repair the laceration.

Jackson (1981) highlighted the whole problem of childhood injuries from glass and pointed out that most of the severe lesions could be prevented by the use of safety glass. Safety glass is laminated and is only about 1.8 times more expensive than the ordinary variety. As yet there are no legal requirements for buildings to have safety glass, only recommendations in codes of practice.

The health visitor is in the ideal situation to see unsafe glass while visiting the home and to suggest that safety glass is used instead.

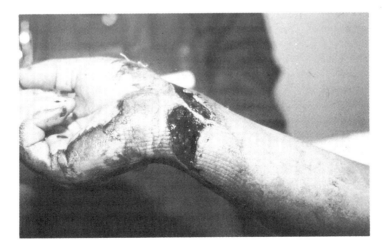

Figure 5.3   Upper limb injuries from a fall onto non-safety glass

Horse Riding Accidents

Horse riding is a common leisure pursuit in children, particularly in girls around puberty. Indeed, horse riding accidents are one of the few types of accident that are more common in girls than boys (Baker, 1973; Nixon et al, 1981), with the peak incidents in 10- to 14-year-old girls. In the UK there are a few deaths from horse riding each year, usually from severe head injuries, but these do not usually reach double figures.

The most common cause of injury is a fall, accounting for just under half of the injuries seen, which may be head injuries, limb fractures and occasionally spinal injuries. Some children are crushed by horses falling on them, and horses also sometimes bite and butt children, kick them and tread on their feet.

Many accidents to children on horseback are caused by inexperience on the part of the rider, particularly when the horse is startled in traffic; injury during competitions is rare. Good supervision and teaching are therefore important in prevention, as is matching the horse and his rider. Good head protection is vital in preventing serious head injury and the importance of wearing of such protection cannot be over-emphasised: in April 1984 a new British Standard (BS 6473) for protective hats for riders was introduced.

Playground Injuries

The dangers for children in playgrounds were highlighted in 1975 by Illingworth et al. She studied children with a variety of playground injuries and found that fractures were three times more common in this group than in attendees at Accident and Emergency Departments as a whole. In South Glamorgan, about one in 50 hospital attendances is due to injuries sustained in a playground. However, only a very few children die in playground accidents: Nixon et al

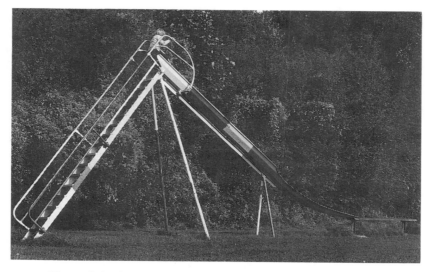

Figure 5.4   Old-fashioned and often dangerous children's slide

(1981) in Australia found that 14 deaths occurred in Brisbane over a five-year period during play and recreation.

The design of playground equipment and the severity and type of accident may be linked. Falls from slides may be severe, especially from the old-fashioned type, where children climb a ladder to a platform 10 or more feet from the ground (Figure 5.4). If the slide follows a contour of a hill or mound (Figure 5.5), there is just as much fun for the children, and a much smaller drop should a mishap occur. Similarly, severe falls can occur from climbing frames: it is just as much fun playing horizontally as vertically, and much less far to fall.

Severe impact injuries can occur from swings made of metal or wood, and trauma can be reduced if they are made of rubberised plastic or, indeed, an old tyre instead. Roundabouts of poor design may trap limbs and cause other significant injuries, and old types, such as the 'witches hat', should not be installed. The nurse in the community, particularly the health visitor, has an important role in persuading the leisure department of the local council to install safe and interesting play equipment.

The playground surface has a bearing on the severity of injuries to children falling onto it. Concrete is twice as hard as grass and 10 times as hard as sand, but there are problems with using sand because of dog and cat fouling. The most satisfactory impact-absorbing surfaces commercially available are a granular bark compound or a specially prepared, rubberised surface.

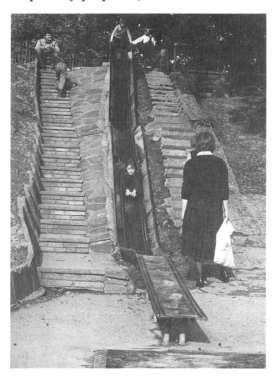

Figure 5.5 Safe children's slide following the contour of a hill

Baby and Child Transport Systems

Babies and young children spend much of their time in perambulators, pushchairs and carrycots. These sites are not without danger, and although it is difficult to estimate the size of the problem, the Home Accident Surveillance System (HASS), which is based on data collected from patients who attend Accident and Emergency Departments, has listed a number of types of accident associated with these modes of transport in 20 hospitals in 1986 (HASS, 1986). There were 112 cases of injury involving a pram, 109 a pushchair, 86 a baby buggy and 21 a carry cot. Three-hundred-and-thirteen children were injured in baby walkers, emphasising the danger of this type of apparatus.

The Consumer Association Report published in the magazine *Which?* in 1986 suggests that of a total of 22 types of pushchair and baby buggy, only four did not have some safety problems. Faults in design included problems with the brakes and brake levers, safety locks, waist straps and crotch straps, and with wheels shearing off.

In a previous report the Consumer Association (1983) noted a number of design faults on pushchairs. Typical were problems with swivelling wheels when only one wheel was fitted with a brake, so that the pushchair could swing around and tip the child out. It was recommended that Government regulations should require buggies with swivelling front wheels to have linked brakes on both back wheels so that one brake could not be used without the other.

Baby prams and pushchairs have been covered by British Standards Institution Regulations since 1979. When parents consult midwives or health visitors about buying a pram or pushchair they should be told to buy only those that are covered by British Standard BS 4792. This standard, modified in 1986, has rectified this and a number of similar faults by law. This standard stipulates that brakes should be able to hold a 15 kg child on a 9 in. slope and that swivel-wheeled pushchairs should have linked brakes on both back wheels. The pushchair should be stable enough not to tip over on a 12 in. slope, and should not have finger traps. Pushchairs should have automatic safety locks and harness attachment points, and the harness should have shoulder straps as well as crotch and waist straps. If the buggy is not fitted with this kind of restraint, a separate safety harness, which complies with British Safety Standard BS 3785, should be fitted. The harness should be adjustable to fit closely and comfortably, so that the child cannot wriggle out underneath it. The fastening should be easy to undo but child-proof.

In addition to these regulations there are other safety points that should be brought to the parent's attention. For instance, accidents occur when hooks and bags for carrying shopping are placed on pushchair handles, which can cause the pushchair to tip over. Accidents also occur when the pushchair is left unattended with the brake off, if the pushchair is used to carry more than one child or if a dog is tied to a stationary pushchair: even if the brake has been applied an accident can result if the dog bolts. The footrest of a pushchair should be adjustable so that small children can rest their feet on it. Ideally, there should be a guard behind the legs to stop older children from hooking their feet behind the footrest and trailing them on the ground, which can result in broken bones.

Pushchairs should not be used for babies under six months old, unless the backrest inclines at an angle of more than 135°. A reclining pushchair should not be used at all unless the child is harnessed securely to prevent the child sliding backwards and out of the pushchair when going up over a high kerb.

Baby Walkers

Baby walkers are becoming increasingly popular. This may be because their use precipitates a pre-ambulatory child taking the long awaited 'first step' or because they afford the child an element of independence which the parents welcome. Alongside their increasing popularity, however, has appeared an increase in accidents arising from their use. In 1977 there were 77 reported accidents which involved baby walkers whereas this had risen to 258 by 1984 (HASS, 1986).

Gleadhill et al (1987) and Whittington (1984) note that it is usually the case that accidents involving baby walkers occur when the child is left unattended or where the environment is such that the child can propel the walker over a step or stairs. The resulting injuries range from head injuries to thermal injuries which occur when the baby walker topples over near hot appliances or an unprotected fire.

The British Standards Institution recommends that a safety warning in permanent, bold lettering be placed on the baby walker – WARNING: NEVER LEAVE YOUR BABY ALONE IN THIS WALKER. However, Gleadhill et al (1987) also report that there is currently no obligation on the part of designers or manufacturers of baby walkers to comply with these recommendations and that few models do so.

Health visitors are ideally placed when visiting the family to note whether a baby walker is being used and to offer advice which would be specific to the needs of the family. A publicity campaign extolling the dangers of baby walkers could be recommended but the effects of this are likely to be as equivocal as other health education campaigns (Minchom et al, 1984). However, since current British Standard recommendations are not being adhered to then it is the responsibility of health professionals to ensure that this is brought to the attention of manufacturers and appropriate national and local organisations. (See Chapter 15.)

Sports and Recreational Injuries

All forms of sport and recreation have some risk associated with them. Office of Population Censuses and Surveys figures (OPCS, 1986) show that in 1982 13 children aged up to 14 years died during sports and leisure activities, including cricket, karting, mountain walking, fishing and athletics. This risk can be reduced by sensible supervision and other safety measures. For instance, hill and mountain climbing expeditions need careful supervision by experienced guides and teachers if disasters are to be prevented. Similarly, it is dangerous to play rugby with teams of different ages and ability as serious neck injuries can lead to paraplegia. Unfortunately, there has been little research on the risks of various sports, in particular on whether rugby or soccer is the more dangerous for boys.

The whole ethos of preventing injuries to children during sport and recreation is difficult. Clearly children cannot be protected from all risks associated with recreational activities, which are important for physical and personality development. On the other hand, children should not be exposed to unnecessary risks. There are few recreational activities for children that do not have some risk, but in most cases the risks can be reduced by sensible precautions.

References

Avery J G (1980) The safety of children in cars. *Practitioner*, **224**: 816–821.

Baker H M (1973) Horse play: survey of accidents with horses. *British Medical Journal*, **3**: 532–534.

Backett E M and Johnson A M (1959) Social patterns of road accidents to children. *British Medical Journal*, **1**: 409.

British Standards Institution (1985) Safety Requirements for Baby Walking Frames. Standard BS 4648. London: British Standards Institution.

Christopherson E R (1977) Children's behaviour during automobile accidents. *Pediatrics*, **60**: 69–74.

Consumer Association (1983) Back Seat Safety. July: 317.

Consumer Association (1984) Childrens' Car Safety Restraints. June: 285.

Gleadhill D N S, Robson W J, Cudmore R E and Turnock R R (1987) Baby walkers . . . time to take a stand. *Archives of Diseases in Childhood*, **62**: 491–494.

HMSO (1980) *Road Accidents Great Britain 1983*. London: HMSO.

Home Accident Surveillance System, An Analysis of Domestic Accidents to Children (1982) London: Department of Trade.

Home Accident Surveillance System 1977–1985. London, Consumer Safety Unit. Department of Trade and Industry, 1986.

Illingworth C M (1985) BMX compared with ordinary bicycle accidents. *Archives of Diseases in Childhood*, **60**: 461–464.

Illingworth C M, Brennan P, Jay A, Al-Rawif E R and Collier M (1975) 200 injuries caused by playground equipment. *British Medical Journal*, **4**: 332–334.

Jackson R H (1981) Lacerations from glass in childhood. *British Medical Journal*, **283**(6302): 1310–1312.

Lauer E, White W C and Lauer B A (1982) Dog bites: a neglected problem in accident prevention. *American Journal of Diseases in Childhood*, **136**(3): 702–704.

Minchom P E, Sibert J R, Newcombe R G and Bowley M A (1984) Does health education prevent accidents? *Postgraduate Medical Journal*, **60**: 260–262.

Nixon, J, Pearn J and McGarn F (1981) Horse riding accidents in childhood. *Safety in Childhood*, **14**(4): 22–24. Melbourne: Accident Prevention Foundation of Australia.

Nixon J, Pearn J and Wilkey I (1981) Deaths during play: a study of playground and recreation deaths in children. *British Medical Journal*, **283**: 410.

OPCS (1986) *Fatal Accidents Occurring During Sporting and Leisure Activities*, DH4 84/3. London: OPCS.

Page M (1985) *Child Safety and Housing: Draft for Discussion*. London: Child Accident Prevention Trust.

Road Accidents in Great Britain 1983 HMSO, London.

Routledge D A, Repetto-Wright R and Hawarth C I (1974) The exposure of young children to accident risk as pedestrians. *Ergonomics*, **17**: 457–480.

Sandel S (1975) *Children in Traffic*. London: Eleck.

Schertz R G (1976) Restraint systems for the prevention of injury to children in automobile accidents. *American Journal of Public Health*, **66**: 451.

Sibert J R, Maddox G B, and Brown M (1981) Childhood accidents: an endemic of epidemic proportions. *Archives of Disease in Childhood*, **56**: 225–234.

Speigel C M and Linderman F (1977) Children can't fly: a program to prevent morbidity and mortality from window falls. *American Journal of Public Health*, **68**: 1143–1147.

Sunderland R (1984) Dying young in traffic. *Archives of Diseases in Childhood*, **59**: 754–757.

Transport and Road Research Laboratory (1979) *The Protection of Children in Cars*, TRRL Leaflet 345. London: TRRL.

Whittington C (1984) *Accidents Involving Baby Walkers*. London: Safety Research Section, Consumer Research Unit.

Recommended Reading

Consumer Association (1990) Child Safety in Cars. May: 290.

County Road Safety Officers Association (1984) *A Highway Code for Children*. Worcester: CRSOA.

Devlin B (1984) Which should you choose? *Nursing Times Community Outlook*, July 11: 248–250.

Health Education Council and the Scottish Health Education Group, in association with the BBC. *Play it Safe. A Guide to Preventing Children's Accidents*. London: HEC/SHEG.

Root J (1983) *Play without Pain*, Melbourne: Child Accident Prevention Foundation of Australia.

Useful Addresses

British Standards Institution
2 Park Street
London W1N 4DE
Tel 071 629 9000

Department of Trade and Industry
Consumer Safety Unit
10–18 Victoria Street
London SW1
Tel 071 215 7877

Chapter 6
First Aid for the Injured Child
Roger Evans

First aid consists of the application of basic medical knowledge with common sense in an emergency situation, using whatever equipment is to hand. While this applies to the immediate treatment of emergencies in either adults or children, it should be borne in mind that the latter will need an even more calm, gentle and considerate approach.

There are certain basic principles that are important to the successful management of an emergency situation and which are entirely based on common sense.

1. Do not panic. Certain situations, for instance facial injuries in a child who has been involved in a road traffic accident may appear shocking due to the distortion produced by fractures, soft tissue swelling and profuse bleeding. The child, if conscious, will certainly be greatly distressed and any atmosphere of panic the helper engenders will heighten this, as well as paralysing the carer as far as effective action is concerned. A health-care professional will have the medical knowledge to cope with the protection of the child's airway, which is the major problem. So, keep cool.
2. Make sure the situation you are about to enter is safe for any helpers present. If a child has collapsed in a gas-filled room, do not immediately rush in to begin artificial ventilation as you are likely also to be overcome by fumes. The supply of the gas should be cut off, at the source if possible, and doors and windows opened to clear the air before entering.
3. Get your priorities right. With an electrocuted child the first priority is to ascertain whether or not he is breathing and his heart beating. The fact that he has burns is of secondary importance and these should not be treated immediately; cardiopulmonary resuscitation (CPR), if necessary, is the first priority. In situations in which there are multiple casualties, those children with airway problems should be attended to before those who are bleeding severely. The child who has minor injuries may well be distressed and crying, which will naturally draw one's attention, but it is the silent unconscious child who needs help most urgently.
4. Do not be over-ambitious. Treatment should be kept within the bounds of competence and be realistic given the situation and circumstances. Medical advice should be summoned if there is a question about any aspect of the patient's management.

The Airway

The maintenance of an open airway from mouth to alveoli is of vital importance. Asphyxia secondary to blockage of the airway by blood-clots, vomit or the sagging tongue is the most common avoidable cause of death in the unconscious patient.

A child who has suffered a head or facial injury is likely to have an impairment of consciousness. If he is lying on his back, his tongue can sag backwards to occlude the airway. Furthermore, injuries to the face cause bleeding from the inside of the nose and mouth, and blood originating from this area can coagulate and, owing to absence of the gag reflex, accumulate in the pharynx and block the airway. The same thing can, of course, occur when the stomach contents are vomited and not completely expelled. It is vital that the airway is opened by extending the patient's neck and clearing any debris out of the mouth and pharynx. A portable sucker, if available, can be employed to good effect clearing the area beyond the reach of the fingers.

The normal manoeuvre of opening the airway by extending the neck and holding it in that position by supporting the head at the nape of the neck and the brow may be used in adolescents. However, in younger children and infants care must be taken not to hyperextend the neck because the cartilaginous rings in the wall of the trachea are not yet well formed and hyperextension can cause the trachea to kink. In infants an extended position may be maintained by supporting the child's head with a soft towel placed beneath the nape of the neck.

The patient, having had his airway cleared, and provided he is now breathing adequately, must be lain on his side in the three-quarter-prone (recovery or coma) position. If possible, he should be tilted slightly head down so that any blood drains down and out rather than into the pharynx.

When the child arrives in hospital his airway will be cleared using suction, which is best applied with the tongue being held forward with a laryngoscope blade so that the illuminated pharynx can be visualised while debris is being removed. Then, if necessary, an endotracheal tube can be inserted and the patient's breathing assisted mechanically.

Bleeding

The sight of blood naturally distresses many adults, and children are at least as likely to be upset by it. A small amount of blood can make an impressive mess, particularly if it has been allowed to drip into and mix with water, as when a cut hand is put under a running tap. Scalp wounds, for instance, which appear to have covered the patient's face with blood, can, when cleaned, be seen to be in fact quite small.

However, these facts notwithstanding, it is always important to staunch bleeding as soon as possible, and in the vast majority of cases this can be accomplished by direct pressure over the wound. Direct pressure means exactly what it says – a clean, preferably sterile, dressing is placed over the wound and held there either by a firm bandage, by the person rendering assistance, or even by the patient himself. This firm pressure applied over the cut vessels reduces the amount of blood flowing from them and makes it easier for blood clots to form. Where practicable (e.g. with a wound to the hand) the injured part should be raised above the level of the heart as this also helps to reduce the blood loss. Care must be taken to ensure that any foreign bodies, e.g. glass, are not present when applying direct pressure to a wound. When foreign bodies are present a ring pad should be applied.

While it is reasonable enough to wash away gently any superficial dirt or grit in the wound, keeping the injury under a gently running tap is counter-productive as this only flushes away any small blood clots that are forming.

Tourniquets are generally unnecessary, as bleeding can usually be controlled by direct pressure. If, however, this form of control proves to be impossible, as perhaps when a foot has been traumatically amputated, the tourniquet should be applied as low down the limb as possible and the patient hospitalised urgently.

Where an amputation has occurred it is always worth while bringing the severed limb or digit in with the patient, preferably wrapped in a sterile towel and kept cool, in the hope that repair will be possible.

Should the patient have suffered a penetrating wound (e.g. to the abdomen) and the instrument is in situ, it should be left where it is firmly embedded and no attempt made to remove it. The implement should be supported on either side by padding to ensure that it moves as little as possible during the patient's transfer to hospital, thus minimising the possibility of further damage.

Nose bleeds are very common in childhood, occurring both spontaneously and secondary to trauma. When the bleeding is spontaneous it usually originates from a small group of dilated blood vessels high up in the nasal passages and if it occurs persistently these will need to be cauterised. The treatment of the acute episode is to sit the child down and make him lean forward, so that the blood trickles out of the nostrils rather than going into the back of the throat. The soft part of the nose should then be gently squeezed, pressure being maintained steadily for about 10 to 15 minutes. When the bleeding has stopped the pressure should be released; the nose should not then be blown as this will merely dislodge the clot and bleeding will restart.

Burns and Scalds

Whatever the cause of the injury, e.g. flames, boiling water, etc., the end result is the same – damage to the skin plus, depending on the amount of heat, damage to the subcutaneous tissues to a varying depth. Burns are of two kinds:

1. Superficial (first and second degree, or partial thickness).
2. Deep (third degree, or full thickness).

Superficial burns are normally identified by the clinical features of pain, erythema, swelling and perhaps some blistering. Deep burns can show all of these features plus charring of the skin and loss of sensation over the burnt areas.

Superficial burns will heal well with minimal treatment, but deep burns usually require skin grafting, and even then will scar badly. The immediate treatment consists of cooling the affected part, e.g. putting a burnt hand in a bowl of cool, clean water, and then, when the pain has eased, covering the burnt area with a light, clean (preferably sterile) dressing. Burnt clothing should be removed only in hospital as it is often stuck to the underlying skin, although clothing that is soaked with boiling water or a corrosive chemical must be taken off immediately. The dead skin, which forms blisters, must initially be allowed to remain in place as it protects the underlying tissue from infection, which is a major problem in burns and accounts for a high percentage of deaths.

Fracture, Sprains and Dislocations

Fractures in children are usually of the variety known as greenstick, in which, because it is less brittle, the child's bone tends to buckle and kink rather than shatter in the way an adult's does. The cardinal features of a fracture are bony tenderness over the fracture site, swelling, immobility and pain on passive movement. Where a fracture is significantly displaced there may also be a deformity of the limb, and a late sign of a fracture is bruising to the area.

Sprains, which are common at the ankle and wrist, occur where there is stretching and tearing of the ligaments surrounding the joint. Sprains can often be difficult to differentiate from fractures as there can be severe swelling, immobility and pain on passive movement; a distinguishing feature, however, is the absence of bony tenderness. If there is any doubt, the injury should be treated as a fracture and the limb immobilised.

Dislocations present with many of the same features as are found with fractures but, of course, they occur only at joints. The most commonly dislocated joints are those of the fingers, while the large joint most often involved is the shoulder.

The treatment of a fracture consists of support and immobilisation. A good general rule is that all fractures of the upper limb (including the shoulder girdle) can be supported and immobilised by strapping the injured limb to the chest using a sling and body bandages. Fractures of the lower limb can be similarly fixed by strapping the injured and uninjured limbs together, preferably with well-padded splints that extend to cover the joints above and below the fracture. Where possible, e.g. with a fracture of the hand, the fracture should be supported above the level of the heart in a high sling, which will minimise the extent of the swelling. For this reason also, fractures of the lower limb should be kept elevated rather than allowed to drop.

It is important to remember that where a splint has been applied and bandaged in place, the circulation in the distal part of the child's limb should be checked regularly (every 10 minutes) in order to ensure that the support is not becoming too tight. This tightness will occur as bleeding from the fracture causes swelling in the area beneath the splint, which, if it produces restriction of the blood flow in the limb can result in permanent damage.

Where a fracture is severely displaced there may be a temptation to 'adjust' the limb. Such manoeuvres are only required exceedingly rarely as emergency procedures and almost invariably should wait until the child is in hospital, where the manipulation can be carried out under general anaesthesia. While many fractures, particularly those of the limbs, will subsequently be immobilised in a plaster cast, some require very little treatment. For instance, a fractured clavicle will only require a sling (the old figure-of-eight bandage is useless) while with some fractures, e.g. those of the fingers, immobilisation for more than four or five days is positively to be avoided as it produces stiffness in the joints, which can subsequently be difficult to relieve.

Sprains are best treated with a cool compress, rest and elevation. They can be supported temporarily with a crêpe or Tubigrip bandage, but if the precise diagnosis is uncertain, they should be regarded as fractures, treated as such and referred on for consideration for X-ray.

Dislocations are much less common than sprains or fractures but are just as painful. They should be supported (e.g. in a broad arm sling for a shoulder dislocation) and only reduced in hospital under a general anaesthetic. Attempts to reduce these injuries shortly after they have occurred, under the mistaken belief that they are more easily reduced early on, are to be deplored as this can cause severe and permanent damage.

When treating an injured child the possibility that the injury may, in the occasional case, have a *non-accidental* aetiology must be remembered. While there is nothing to be gained by alienating every parent by tactless questioning, the health-care professional is quite entitled to expect reasonable and believable answers to polite questions about how the injury was sustained.

The Unconscious Child

When faced with an unconscious child the immediate priority is to safeguard his airway, as discussed previously; precise diagnosis can wait until a clear airway has been established. Having dealt with any urgent problems, a history should be taken from relatives, friends or bystanders, gleaning all possible information and not forgetting to ask about access to drugs and other toxic substances. The patient should be examined carefully, noting his level of consciousness (Figure 6.1) and any change in this, together with the rate, rhythm and volume of the pulse (*See* pages 74–75). Bruising, external bleeding or other evidence of trauma, particularly bleeding from the nose or ears or, perhaps, the leakage of

Fully conscious	Wide awake and responding
Drowsy	Appears lightly asleep but is easily woken by minimal stimuli, e.g. pinching his ear lobe gently. The child can answer basic questions, e.g. name, address and date
Stuporous	Appears deeply asleep and only responds poorly to strong stimuli, e.g. rubbing his sternum with your knuckles. Resents being woken and gives a poor response to any questions
Comatose	Totally unresponsive

Figure 6.1   Levels of consciousness

cerebrospinal fluid (CSF) from these orifices, may be seen. The child's temperature should be taken and rashes noted. The child may be wearing a medic-alert bracelet or locket, which could give a clue to the reason for the unconscious episode. The pupils should be examined noting whether or not they are unresponsive or unequal.

When the child is taken to hospital, he should be accompanied by all the information collected.

Figure 6.2 shows the common causes of unconsciousness in childhood. There are many others that are not listed, but the vast majority of the unconscious children likely to be encountered will have one of the problems described below.

Head Injuries	
Post-ictal states	e.g. secondary to febrile convulsions and grand-mal fits
Poisoning	e.g. drugs, alcohol, seeds and berries, domestic and cosmetic preparations
Meningitis/encephalitis	
Diabetes	as a complication of insulin treatment

Figure 6.2   Common causes of unconsciousness in childhood

Cardiopulmonary Resuscitation (CPR)

Cardiopulmonary resuscitation in children, as in adults, aims to keep the vital organs, particularly the brain, oxygenated until the heart can be restarted in its normal rhythm. The principles are basically the same but are modified to suit the smaller, less mature frame of the child and to take account of the fact that he normally has a more rapid pulse rate than does an adult. A step by step guide to CPR is as follows:

1. Confirm that a cardiac arrest has occurred (see Figure 6.3).
2. Quickly lay the child on a firm surface.
3. Begin artificial ventilation and external cardiac massage.

The techniques of these two procedures and the detail of how to implement them, are now described, both for solo resuscitation and resuscitation with an assistant undertaking one of the tasks.

Mouth-to-Mouth Ventilation

Open the child's airway, being careful not to hyperextend the neck, and make a tight seal around his mouth (or mouth and nose in a baby) with your lips. Pinch the nostrils closed and then blow into the airway with sufficient pressure to make the chest rise – this can be observed out of the corner of the eye. Initially, give

The child is unconscious

Breathing is absent

There is no palpable pulse (use the femoral artery)

The child is pale and cyanosed

The pupils are dilated and do not react to light

Figure 6.3   Signs of cardiac arrest

five rapid deep breaths to 'freshen up' the air in the child's lungs, then settle into a steady rhythm of between 20 and 30 breaths per minute.

External Cardiac Massage

In adolescents cardiac massage is carried out using similar techniques to those used for adults, making modifications given that the subject is smaller. The heel of one hand is placed over the lower half of the sternum with the arm held stiff and vertical, the resuscitator's shoulder being directly above the patient's sternum. The sternum is depressed about 3–4 cm (1–1½ in.) in a smooth, sharp movement, and then, after a short pause, pressure is relaxed and the sternum allowed to spring back into its normal position.

In infants the sternum usually only needs to be depressed about 2 cm, and this can be achieved with light pressure from only two or three fingers. Alternatively, the baby's torso may be gripped with both hands, the thumbs meeting at the sternum and the finger tips at the thoracic spine; the thumbs can then be used to depress the sternum for the required distance.

For infants and small children a rate of 120 compressions/minute should be used; for a five-year-old 100/minute is acceptable and for older children 80/minute.

When in the fortunate position of having two resuscitators, one can ventilate the patient while the other massages the heart. Under these circumstances, work on a one-to-five (1:5) ratio, i.e. the child receives one deep breath in the gap after each fifth cardiac compression, the heart massage being uninterrupted. If alone, work on a two-to-fifteen ratio (2:15), the child receiving two deep breaths for every 15 cardiac compressions.

Chapter 7
Head Injuries
J R Sibert   Donna Mead

Head injury is a common clinical problem. Many children are admitted to hospital each year for observation in case they develop an intracranial haemorrhage; however, the vast majority recover and are well afterwards. In a study carried out in Wales between 1974 and 1981, of 28 701 children admitted to hospital, only 35 (1 in 820) developed an intracranial haemorrhage (Sainsbury and Sibert, 1984).

Children may injure their heads in many ways. Pedestrian road traffic accidents are the cause of many serious head injuries and, indeed, they represent a major cause of death and handicap. Equally, children in cars may injure their heads, especially if they are not in adequate seat restraints. Bicycle accidents account for a surprisingly large number of head injuries, often associated with facial lacerations and abrasions: in South Glamorgan alone approximately one in 500 boys was admitted to hospital in 1983 following a head injury when riding a bicycle. Serious head injury may also be found in cases of child abuse, where subdural haematoma is a sinister complication. More commonly children injure their heads by falling from windows or trees or playground equipment while playing at school or outside. Falling down the stairs is a particular problem with toddlers.

Complications

The major complications of head injuries are skull fracture, convulsions, intracranial haemorrhage and permanent brain damage. Other problems include cerebrospinal leaks, particularly CSF rhinorrhoea, facial and scalp lacerations and blood in the middle ear.

A skull fracture by itself is not usually a major problem of management; however, it is an indication that the injury was severe enough to break the cranial bones. Infection may enter the meninges through a skull fracture and associated lacerations.

Convulsions are an infrequent complication of head injury; they may occur in a child already liable to fits, may be an indication of severe brain injury or may be a short-lived phenomenon, which may not be repeated. A child who has a fit should be assessed by a doctor and observed in hospital.

Intracranial haemorrhage is the most worrying complication of head injury and is the reason why so many children are admitted to hospital each year for observation. Children may develop an extradural or subdural haematoma: both may be acute or chronic. Intracranial haemorrhage may be suspected from the signs and symptoms of increasing intracranial pressure or from localising signs. When diagnosed, urgent evacuation of the haematoma is needed.

Severe and permanent brain damage is a rare but very significant complication of major head injuries, particularly because of the impact it has on the child and family. Few people who have witnessed him can forget the brain-injured child with severe spastic quadriplegia, who takes all the family's energy, to the detriment of the other siblings. The true incidence of severe permanent brain damage following head injury is unknown; however, one in four children with post-traumatic intracranial haemorrhage is subsequently found to be significantly brain damaged. Brain damage following a head injury does not always have its basis in the direct effects of the injury, e.g. bleeding. If the child becomes unconscious or has an associated jaw injury, airway obstruction may result; this leads to difficulty in maintaining an adequate airflow to the lungs and can result in hypoxia, which is itself a significant cause of brain damage.

Presentation of Head Injuries

Children with head injuries may have many symptoms. Clearly unconsciousness always causes alarm and is another pointer to the severity of the injury. Vomiting may also be a significant symptom of raised intracranial pressure, although it may just reflect a particular reaction to stress. Diplopia should never be ignored and may follow pressure on the VIth intracranial nerve from increased intracranial pressure and direct trauma. Headache is a much more variable and less significant symptom, unless the headache continues to increase in severity.

CSF leaks from the ear and nose and bleeding from the ear should be considered a serious symptom; bleeding from the nose, however, is usually the result of direct trauma.

A boggy scalp haematoma is an important pointer to intracranial haemorrhage. One of the most important physical signs of localising intracranial haemorrhage is the dilated pupil: pupil size and reaction are a vital part of the nursing observation of head injuries.

A child who appears fully alert and who denies a period of unconsciousness should have this story confirmed by a witness if possible. It may be that the child cannot remember that he has lost consciousness. Amnesia for events leading up to a head injury may indicate that the level of injury is more severe than in patients whose recollections are clear. It is important, therefore, that all questions about the accident are put to the child, provided that he is able to respond, and that the responses are confirmed by a witness.

Management of Head Injuries

First Aid

The first task when confronted with a child with a severe head injury is to maintain his airway and prevent inhalation of vomit. There is no doubt that many children suffer brain damage after a head injury because of hypoxia due to an obstructed airway. In the Accident and Emergency Department or health centre, a plastic airway or endotracheal intubation with a cuffed tube will obviously be the most effective way of maintaining the airway. Away from facilities, when one is confronted with a child with an obstructed airway who has a head injury, a cursory examination should be made for obvious injuries to the spine. If such injuries are present, the child should be kept on his back with the head and neck carefully extended. In the absence of spinal injuries the child should be placed on his side and the tongue brought forward either by gravity or with the fingers.

Assessment in the Accident and Emergency Department

When seen in the Accident and Emergency Department a head-injured child should be assessed for: the cause of the injury, and, in particular, the area of the head affected and the forces involved; whether or not a period of unconsciousness or drowsiness followed the injury and, if it did, how long it lasted; whether or not the child vomited, had a fit or exhibited diplopia; and whether or not there has been any bleeding or CSF loss from the nose or ear. Other injuries, including lacerations, abrasions and dental trauma, should also be assessed. The assessment should include searching for a boggy scalp haematoma and a brief neurological examination, including the pupils and optic fundi. Other problems, such as otitis media, should also be looked for.

There has been much debate in the past on whether or not children with head injuries need to have skull X-rays. Children may develop extradural haematomata without a skull fracture, but the incidence of intracranial haemorrhage is higher in children with a skull fracture than in those without this complication. Intracranial injury is also an indication of the severity of the force of the injury. It is prudent, therefore, for all children with significant head injuries to have a skull X-ray.

The advent of computed axial tomography (CAT) scanning has made the detection of raised intracranial pressure easier. Performing this investigation is now an essential part of the modern management of severe head injuries in children.

Which Children Should We Observe and Which Should We Send Home?

At present, standard practice is to admit for 24-hours' observation all children assessed as having a significant head injury. Head injuries are considered significant if there has been more than momentary unconsciousness, amnesia of the events that preceded the accident, continued drowsiness, vomiting, diplopia, fitting, bleeding from the ear, cerebrospinal fluid leak from the nose, a skull fracture or a boggy scalp haematoma.

Many nurses and doctors have been concerned with the present pattern of head injury observation. The vast majority of these cases come to no harm and, in retrospect, need not have been admitted. However, some children seen soon after injury are discharged home only to be admitted later on developing neurological signs such as dizziness and vomiting. This is of especial relevance with regard to extradural haematoma where, classically, there is a lucid interval, with unconsciousness following the injury, recovery and then increasing drowsiness and physical signs of raised intracranial pressure.

However, is 24-hours' observation needed for safety? Recent work from Glasgow has suggested that, in adults, a more limited observation period may be sufficient (Jennett and Galbraith, 1979). Sainsbury and Sibert (1984) have looked at post-traumatic intracranial haemorrhage in Wales over an eight-year period, and found that in all the cases of head injury that developed this complication there were clear reasons for continued admission after a six-hour period of observation. They suggest that many children may be observed in hospital for a shorter period and, if well and symptom-free, can be safely discharged home with clear advice on and specific instructions for action if complications do occur. (Figure 7.1). Clearly children with major symptoms or signs such as fitting or unconsciousness on presentation need longer periods of observation.

If this policy were adopted, it can be seen that the only children admitted following head injury would be those for whom neurological complications were a very real probability. Such a policy may have the advantage that Accident and Emergency staff, in knowing that discharge will take place after six hours if no neurological signs are present, will be extremely vigilant in observing the child during this period, thus averting the few occasions when children are discharged home only to develop an intracranial haemorrhage later. In the future the most suitable place for observation may not necessarily be the ward, but might be a specially equipped and staffed part of the Accident and Emergency Department, set aside for the observation and treatment of children.

Your child has received an injury to the head. A careful examination has been made, and no signs of any serious complication have been found.
It is expected that recovery will be rapid. However, if any vomiting, dizziness, headache, double vision or excessive drowsiness are noticed, you should telephone the hospital at once.

Figure 7.1   Sample discharge instructions after head injury

Observations and Management

Proper neurological observation is crucial because of the small number of children who develop extradural haematomata following a head injury. Such children usually have a history of losing consciousness at the time of the injury, then being lucid, and later becoming drowsy, before developing neurological signs and again losing consciousness. A history containing these details, however, is not always available. For this reason all children who are admitted to hospital following a head injury must be constantly observed for the following:

1.   Level of consciousness. This includes determining whether the child is alert, drowsy but easy to rouse, or drowsy but difficult to rouse. Also, the

child should be assessed for disorientation and confusion. The parents should be encouraged to assist in this assessment as the child is more likely to respond to his mother's familiar voice than to a stranger's. The mother is also the person who will know best the familiar phrases to which the child is likely to respond.

2. The size of the child's pupils and their reaction to light. Under normal circumstances the pupils should be equal in size and react briskly (by constricting) when exposed to a bright light, both pupils responding in this way to a light shone in one eye alone. Sluggish reaction to light and dilation of the pupil indicates raised intracranial pressure.

3. The power of movement in all four limbs. If the child is conscious, this involves assessing whether or not he can move his limbs spontaneously and equally on command to do so. In the case of the unconscious child, it involves noting how the limbs respond to painful stimuli.

4. Vital signs such as pulse rate, respiratory rate and blood pressure. Initially if there is cerebral hypoxia as a result of the injury, the respirations will increase in rate and depth. As the intracranial pressure continues to rise, however, a point may arise when the cerebral hypoxia depresses the respiratory centre. The respiration rate will then start to fall until, in the terminal stages, respiration becomes slow, shallow and irregular.

   As intracranial pressure increases, blood pressure rises as a result of the vasomotor centre's response to hypoxia; it is an inappropriate attempt to improve blood flow. At the same time there is a fall in the pulse rate, which occurs in response to the increase in blood pressure.

5. As the intracranial pressure rises the child will become more irritable and fractious. He may vomit or complain of a headache. It is important that the nurse is able to communicate with the child in terms that he can understand. The mother should be asked which words the child uses for pain, feeling sleepy or feeling sick. For example, pain to many children is a 'baddy'; they may express the need to sleep as 'going bye byes'; feeling sick might become 'picky Mummy', and so on.

A chart that helps to monitor patient behaviour as well as objective neurological signs is useful. The Glasgow Coma Scale (Allan, 1984a,b, 1986) and the paediatric coma scale (Allan and Culne-Seymour, 1989), which is an adaptation of this, is recommended for this purpose. This chart has the advantage also of doing away with the need for words like 'stupor' or 'semi-comatose', which may mean different things to different people.

It should be remembered that patients with multiple injuries should have appropriate attention paid to other sites of trauma.

If there is any change in the child's neurological status or if a fit occurs, a full medical assessment is needed.

In keeping with the philosophy for caring for children in hospital, the parents should be encouraged to stay with the child at this time.

As with all injured children, the causes of the accident should be explored for possible action to prevent a similar occurrence.

Management of Complications of Head Injury

The management of an isolated skull fracture is not usually a problem, except when the fracture is associated with lacerations or abrasions. In such cases, infection may enter the meninges, but prophylactic antibiotics will help to prevent this complication. Traumatic perforation of the ear and CSF rhinorrhoea should also have antibiotic protection.

Where convulsions follow a head injury, particular attention should be paid to maintenance of the airway. The convulsions should be stopped with a drug such as diazepam, preferably given intravenously; rectal diazepam is an acceptable alternative. It is unwise to start regular anticonvulsants unless the fits are repeated.

Intracranial haemorrhage will be suspected from the signs and symptoms of raised intracranial pressure, such as vomiting and papilloedema, or by localising signs of the blood clot, such as a dilated fixed pupil or VIth nerve palsy. Diagnosis may be helped by computed tomography of the head. When diagnosed, urgent evacuation of the haematoma is needed to prevent brain damage and death. Burr holes are best drilled by neurosurgeons and if transfer to a specialist centre is essential, it should take place without delay. Appropriately trained medical and nursing escorts are needed. Unnecessary transfers can be avoided by sending the CAT scan by electronic mail to the specialist centre.

Cerebral oedema may complicate severe head injury, especially when there has been associated hypoxia. This may cause further brain damage, and may be treated with the osmotic diuretic mannitol and the steroid dexamethasone.

Long-Term Follow-Up and Rehabilitation

Severe head injuries in children may lead to mental retardation and cerebral palsy. There may be incoordination and difficulty in performing fine tasks. The care of such children, as with all handicapped children, needs the help of a multidisciplinary team, which may include a paediatrician, nurses (especially health visitors), physiotherapists, occupational therapists, speech therapists and teachers. Special educational provision may also be needed.

The burden of a severely brain-damaged child on the family is considerable, and may lead to social complications that may even last for generations. The burden is made more difficult because of the sense of guilt parents sometimes have that they were to blame for the initial accident.

Prevention of Head Injuries

As there are many causes of head injury, there may be many preventive solutions. Many severe head injuries are caused in road traffic accidents, which can best be prevented by better supervision of child pedestrians, environmental road schemes and rear safety belts in cars.

Many children, particularly boys, injure their heads in bicycle accidents, and head protection may reduce the severity of their injuries.

In the *Children Can't Fly* programme in New York (Spiegal and Ludaven,

1977), window falls have been prevented by the provision of free window guards. Their widespread use needs to be advocated.

Finally, the modern management of non-accidental injury should help to prevent severe child abuse, which may cause subdural haematoma and brain damage.

References

Allan D (1984a) Glasgow Coma Scale. *Nursing*, **2**: 668.

Allan D (1984b) Glasgow Coma Scale. *Nursing Mirror*, **158**: 23, 32.

Allan D (1986) Management of the head-injured patient. *Nursing Times*, **82**(25): 36–39.

Allan D and Culne-Seymour C (1989) Paediatric coma scale. *Nursing Times*, **85**(20): 44–45.

Jennett B and Galbraith S L (1979) Head injury and admission policy. *Lancet*, **1**: 552.

Sainsbury C P Q and Sibert J R (1984) How long do we need to observe head injuries in hospital? *Archives of Diseases in Childhood*, **59**: 856–859.

Spiegal G N and Ludaven F C (1977) Children can't fly: a programme to prevent morbidity and mortality from window falls. *American Journal of Public Health*, **67**: 1143–1147.

Recommended Reading

Boylan A and Brown P (1985) Neurological observations. *Nursing Times*, **81**(27): 36–40.

Wood T and Milne P (1988) Head injury to pedal cyclists and the promotion of helmet use in Victoria, Australia. *Accid, Anal and Prev*, **20**: 177–185.

Chapter 8
Eye Injuries
Janet Bott

Ophthalmic injuries in children are a common and serious problem, not only because of the acute effects but also because of the long-term sequelae, which may result in impaired vision, loss of an eye, a disfigured eye or even blindness.

It is extremely difficult to evaluate what a child loses as a result of a damaged eye – lack of depth perception, stereopsis and binocular vision may not significantly affect him in his school work, but there will be certain jobs from which he will be excluded as a result of his handicap. If enucleation is performed early in life, facial asymmetry may occur, resulting in disfigurement.

Common ophthalmic injuries in children are either penetrating, blunt or the result of burns, being either intraocular or extraocular. The causes range from being hit in the eye with a ball and falling on blunt or sharp objects, to lacerations from tree branches, air gun pellets and chemical burns as a result of accidents at home or at school. Crombie (1982) reports that the main cause of eye accidents in children, in order of frequency, are arrows, air gun pellets and assaults with pointed objects. In the description that follows, injuries have been grouped into intraocular and extraocular, with intraocular injuries further divided into penetrating and blunt, and extraocular into penetrating, blunt and burns. In Manchester Royal Eye Hospital, a busy regional referral centre for 4.5 million people, more than half the urgent admissions to the children's ward during 1985 were due to injury, the ratio being 66 boys to 14 girls. This sex difference is consistent with the pattern for the country as a whole, with four males being involved for every one female.

Injuries in Relation to Age and Development

0–1 Year old

The accident that most commonly happens to a child in this age group is falling, either from one level to another or as a result of an adult dropping the child. Should an eye injury occur from an accident of this nature, it is likely to result in a hyphaema or an orbital fracture.

Corneal and conjunctival abrasions may occur as a result of the child hitting himself with toys. Fingernail scratches also are fairly common and are the result of undeveloped motor skills. Siblings may sometimes be responsible for blows and scratches to the eyes of children in this age group.

1–5 Years old

The child is now an adventurous toddler, and as such is at risk from accidents that result in penetrating injuries. These may occur as a result of the child running around while carrying pens or other sharp objects: if he should fall or collide with another person, a penetrating eye injury may result. Children of this age group may also sustain an injury of this nature from running into table corners.

A toddler who plays with pets is likely to receive scratches or bites around the eye, or possibly even lid lacerations, the risk of which is enhanced if the child teases the pet.

The Older Child

It can be seen that many of the eye injuries that occur in children of this age group do so as a result of the inevitable decrease in parental supervision.

Fights are common and may result in orbital fractures and hyphaemas. As the child participates more in sport the risk of sporting injuries increases, the most common type of which results from being hit by a ball. Eye injuries received while at play are commonly due to the injudicious use of catapults and to stone-throwing. Adolescence is the age at which boys take an interest in air rifles and pistols: air gun pellet injuries are, therefore, common at this time.

Initial Examination

Whatever the nature of the eye injury, an initial assessment of both eyes must be made by systematic examination. This procedure should be repeated whenever eye dressings are removed or replaced: in so doing, complications are detected early and progress assessed.

The examination procedure involves inspection of:

1. the lids, for signs of allergy, infection or laceration;
2. the conjunctiva, for chemosis, increased redness and the condition of sutures if present;
3. the cornea for clarity and integrity;
4. the anterior chamber, for depth, hyphaema or hypopyon;
5. the pupil, for size, shape and reaction to light;
6. the iris, for lack of iris pattern and normal sparkle on exposure to light, which may indicate inflammation within the eye;
7. the wound, particularly the suture line for loose sutures of an iris that has prolapsed through the wound;
8. the full range of ocular movements.

The examination is completed by noting any increase in pain or marked loss of vision.

The nurse should remember that the above procedures may constitute a traumatic and frightening experience for the child concerned. If the examination is to be completed successfully, the following simple guidelines should be taken into account:

1.   If possible, ensure that the parents are present.
2.   Adopt a sympathetic but firm approach.
3.   Ensure that the parents know how to hold the child securely.
4.   Take the time beforehand to gain the child's co-operation, as there is nothing to be gained from attempting either an eye examination or dressing with a frightened, struggling child. This is best achieved by providing an adequate explanation and, in the case of the younger child, using distraction techniques. Co-operation is often achieved if play is used as the medium through which explanations are given, for example, allowing the child to perform eye dressings on a doll.

Intraocular Injuries

Intraocular injuries include all those that damage the eye and its internal structure.

Penetrating Injuries

Foreign Bodies   Intraocular foreign bodies can be high-speed objects, e.g. airgun pellets or fragments of flying glass, metal or wood, that penetrate the globe. An intraocular foreign body must always be suspected after a penetrating injury has occurred, and all cases of penetrating injuries with a history that indicates the possibility of a retained foreign body should be admitted as an emergency. Skull X-rays to enable the foreign body to be located should be taken while the child is in casualty prior to admission. If the foreign body is non-metallic, tomograms and ultrasound are indicated to visualise it.

Complications of Intraocular Foreign Body Injuries.   Infection is a major risk with all penetrating injuries and will require large doses of oral antibiotics for its prevention.

If the foreign body has ruptured one of the blood vessels in the iris, a hyphaema will result. Vitreous haemorrhage will occur if the retinal blood vessels have been damaged.

Cataract formation may occur if the lens metabolism is disturbed.

Metallic foreign bodies can cause severe reactions in the eye and need to be removed as soon as possible. Fragments of copper cause a condition known as chalcosis, which results in the formation of large amounts of pus in the eye. A retained intraocular foreign body of iron causes a local condition in the eye known as siderosis, which results in degeneration and death of tissues within the eye.

Ferrous metallic foreign bodies are removed in theatre with a giant hand magnet. Toxic, non-metallic substances, such as eye lashes, insect stings, caterpillar hairs and wood, and non-ferrous metallic objects have to be removed surgically.

Inert substances, such as silver, gold, glass and plastic, do not usually cause specific reactions and if left may become encapsulated.

With a severely damaged eye, or one that is unresponsive to treatment, the risk that sympathetic ophthalmitis may develop in the other eye must be considered. This is a severe form of uveitis; its cause is unknown but it is thought to be due either to an inflammatory reaction to pigmentary tissue, or possibly to a virus introduced at the time of injury. When sympathetic ophthalmitis occurs the decision as to whether or not to enucleate has to be taken within two weeks of the injury if the inflammatory reaction is to be prevented, because once it has occurred removal of the eye will not halt the progress of the ophthalmitis in the remaining eye. A second medical opinion is usually sought before this decision is made. Sympathetic ophthalmitis usually occurs within eight weeks of the injury, but cases have been reported up to 50 years after the event.

Trauma to Cornea and Sclera

Corneal Abrasions   Corneal abrasions can be caused by contact lenses, finger-nail scratches and foreign bodies such as wind-blown dirt, and result in damage to the epithelial layer of the cornea. This layer has a plentiful supply of free nerve endings, so injury produces extreme pain, lacrimation and photophobia. The diagnosis can be made by staining the cornea with fluorescein and examining the eye with a blue light – the abraded areas will appear green.

A young child with a foreign body in his eye may, depending on his age, need to be admitted for its removal under general anaesthetic. In older, more co-operative children, superficial foreign bodies may be removed in the casualty department with a 21g needle and illuminated magnification.

After removal of any foreign body, treatment by antibiotic ointment is indicated to prevent secondary infection and to act as a lubricant. A mydriatic/cycloplegic agent may be instilled to stop ciliary spasm and thus relieve pain. A pad will be applied.

Lacerations   Corneal and scleral lacerations in children are usually caused by knives, sharp toys and pens. If global penetration is suspected, care must be taken not to exert pressure on the eye as this may cause ocular tissue to prolapse through the wound. The eye is padded and cartella shield (a dome of plastic or metal with holes in it that is used to cover and protect the eye) applied. The child is taken to the operating theatre as soon as possible, where the eye can be examined and the degree of injury assessed and treated.

Once in theatre antitetanus toxoid is given if required, and swabs are taken for culture and sensitivity. The open wound is sutured, and any iris prolapse is incised and repaired, the anterior chamber being reconstituted with either air or saline. Antibiotic drops are instilled and a course of systemic antibiotics prescribed. A sub-conjunctival injection of antibiotics is also given. Finally, the eye is covered with a pad and a bandage applied.

Complications
1. Infection is a major hazard and perhaps the most serious complication. It may be seen either as a discharge from the conjuctiva or as a hypopyon,

which is pus in the anterior chamber shown as a level of creamy white substance obscuring part of the iris.

2. Corneal scarring may lead to loss of vision, and a corneal graft may be indicated later if this occurs. Unfortunately, despite tremendous improvements in graft techniques, corneal grafting does not always restore vision.
3. A shrunken globe may result from loss of ocular tissue at the time of injury.
4. If the eye becomes blind and painful, it may have to be removed.
5. Sympathetic ophthalmitis can occur.

Blunt Injuries

The most common blunt injuries are caused by balls, fists, stones and shuttlecocks.

Hyphaema Hyphaema is the presence of blood in the anterior chamber following haemorrhage of the iris; it may be microscopic or macroscopic. All patients with hyphaema are admitted for bed-rest because of the possibility that a secondary haemorrhage may occur. Other complications of hyphaema include staining of the cornea by red blood cells and secondary glaucoma caused by blockage of the filtration angle.

Bed-rest allows the hyphaema to absorb and reduces the risk of further bleeding. It is maintained for between three and five days or until the clot has dispersed. A pad or cartella shield may be applied. Other treatment may include topical antibiotics to prevent secondary infection. Any raised intraocular pressure will be corrected by reducing the formation of aqueous humour by the administration of a drug that inhibits the formation of the enzyme carbonic anhydrase and thus reduces the rate at which aqueous humour is formed. The same effect can also be achieved by the use of a beta-adrenoceptor blocking drug, e.g. timolol. Surgical intervention may be necessary in severe cases.

Paralysed Iris A common feature of blunt injury is a paralysed iris, referred to as traumatic mydriasis if the pupil is dilated and traumatic miosis if it is constricted. In both cases the pupil does not react to stimulation by light.

Prior to discharge the child's eye should be examined for other complications, such as commotioretina (traumatic disruption of the retina), cataract formation, iridodialysis (separation of the iris from the ciliary body), dislocated lens, vitreous haemorrhage and retinal detachment.

Extraocular Injuries

Penetrating Injuries

Extraocular penetrating injuries are lid lacerations, which may or may not involve the canaliculi. Causes ranges from a severe blow to the eye with resultant tearing, to falling on sharp objects, to dog bites.

Repair of lacerations is a lengthy procedure, which is performed under a general anaesthetic because the lids have to be sutured layer by layer to ensure regularity of the lid margins and alignment of the tarsal plate so that lacrimal secretion and drainage are unimpaired. Torn canaliculi need to be repaired surgically with the insertion of a tube to maintain patency. This tube, which allows free drainage of tears, remains in situ for approximately six weeks until healing has occurred. Tetanus toxoid is given while in the operating theatre; local antibiotic ointment is instilled and a pad applied.

Complications
1. All lid traumas can cause damage to secretory glands, resulting in decreased lacrimation. This can be alleviated in the long term by the instillation of artificial tears.
2. Damage to the levator palpebrae muscle causes ptosis, the inability to elevate the upper eyelid. Surgical techniques may be needed to correct this.

Blunt Injuries

A direct blow to the eye by an object, for example a ball or fist, can cause injuries such as sub-conjunctival haemorrhage and ecchymosis, which usually require no treatment. It can also cause an orbital fracture, which may need treatment.

Orbital fractures can occur in the roof, medial wall or floor of the orbit, the most common place being the orbital floor: this is referred to as a "blow out" fracture. A fracture of the orbital floor can be further complicated by the trapping of the inferior oblique and inferior rectus muscles in the fracture, thus restricting ocular movement. If this occurs, the patient will complain of diplopia on vertical gaze, and surgery is indicated. The muscles are freed and a teflon implant inserted.

Burns

Very few accidents in childhood lead to bilateral blindness, but if this does happen, it is usually the result of an explosion or of acid or alkali burns. Although the most common causes of burn damage to the eyes are radiation and chemicals, damage by heat or from electrical sources may also occur.

Radiation Burns Radiation burns are caused by ultraviolet rays from such sources as sun lamps and arc welding equipment. The child usually presents approximately 10 hours after exposure with pain, redness and gritty sensations in the eyes. The diagnosis is made by staining the cornea with fluorescein: the damaged epithelium will appear green when examined with a blue light.

Treatment includes antibiotic treatment and short-acting cycloplegics.

The eyes are padded for 24 hours and the patient advised to take oral analgesics, as the condition is very painful.

This type of injury is usually seen in older, adolescent children who have access to sun lamps. Admission to hospital is not necessary in such instances, and parents are given advice on how to care for their child at home.

Chemical Burns Chemical burns are caused by acids or alkalis and require immediate treatment. Alkali burns are the more serious because an alkali continues to penetrate the tissue, whereas acid burns the area of contact only and does not tend to penetrate the cornea. With all chemical burns the immediate treatment is irrigation, usually with normal saline, to dilute and flush away any remaining corrosive, thus preventing further damage. Staining of the eye will show any damaged areas.

A child with chemical burns will usually be admitted to hospital for treatment with mydriatic and cycloplegic eye drops and antibiotics. An important complication is symblepharon, which is adhesions between the conjunctiva lining the globe and the conjunctiva lining the eyelids. Severe corneal scarring may also occur and later require corneal grafting. Scarring of the eyelids may cause trichiasis, where the eye lashes turn inwards and scratch the cornea, leading to ulceration if allowed to persist.

Should complications such as blindness, monocular vision or a disfigured eye occur after injury, the effects for the child can be devastating in terms of future employment prospects and physical and psychological consequences. These effects, therefore, are discussed in more detail below.

The Effects of Blindness

Although the number of children who become permanently blind through eye injury is small, the effects on these children are enormous and include separation from family and friends if residential schooling is necessary, and the difficulties involved in mastering new techniques, such as reading braille. Both parents and child can have tremendous problems in adjusting to the handicap. While facilities and support are available for blind children, the tragedy is that any place should be occupied by a child who is blinded by injury.

Temporary blindness or impairment of vision may be due to the nature of the injury, for example bilateral swollen eyelids, corneal abrasions or burns, thus making the eyes painful to open, the instillation of cycloplegic drops to both eyes, or both eyes being padded.

When blindness occurs, reactions may include a fear of moving about alone, unwillingness to participate in ward or family activity for fear of making mistakes and looking foolish, regressive behaviour such as bedwetting, and reactive behaviour such as general apathy and not wanting to get dressed or eat unaided. However, these feelings and fears should gradually disappear as the child begins to learn that he can manage, or when some vision returns. It is important to allow the child to try things for himself and to make mistakes. Bumps and bruises are inevitable, especially if the temporary blindness is likely to last for several weeks. It should be remembered, however, that newly acquired blindness, whether temporary or permanent, will probably be a frightening and upsetting experience for the child. The effects can be minimised by basing nursing actions on the following simple goals:

1.   *Minimise the frightening aspects of blindness/impaired vision*

- Whenever the child is approached the nurse should identify herself by name and state the reason for her presence.

- Make absolutely certain that explanation of procedures is adequate. There is no place for anything less than absolute honesty with a newly blinded child, even if the condition is temporary. This is especially so with regard to procedures that may be painful. It is important that the nurse should talk to the child throughout any procedure.

2. *Minimise the effects of boredom and loneliness.*

- Ensure that the child is able to contact a member of staff should he want to.
- Maintain contacts with the child's school and friends. Taped messages from people the child knows will be welcome.

Make use of learning sources and means of enjoyment e.g. hospital radio, listening to children's programmes on television and audiotaped stories, that do not require sight.

3. *Maintain the level of independence already achieved.* Be patient, allow the child to do those things for himself which he did before the accident – to the extent that this is safe. For example, the nurse should be patient at meal times when the child wants to feed himself. Supervision of meals can be a laborious process, but the time spent will be worth while if it leads to maintaining independence, which will aid in preserving the child's self-esteem. To this end the nurse should remember to make use of the aids available, e.g. bendy straws and non-slip mats.

4. *Ensure that the child's environment remains safe.* The nurse's involvement in this endeavour will depend upon the child's stage development and level of co-operation. The principles of care are those which will safeguard the child from further injury, and to that end, the nurse will ensure adequate supervision whenever necessary.

5. *Ensure that the parents receive support commensurate with the nature of the blindness.* Where blindness is permanent, ensure that parents receive or know where to obtain the necessary guidance and counselling. This should occur as soon as possible so that the parents are aware from the outset that they will receive help and support from organisations such as The Royal National Institute for the Blind (RNIB), the RNIB Education Advisory Service and the Advisory Centre for Education (addresses can be found at the end of this chapter).

Local Education Authorities may know of a peripatetic teacher for the visually handicapped within the child's local area, and the local Social Services department will provide the family with the support of a social worker.

6. *Minimise psychological reactions to blindness.* Periods of regressive and aggressive behaviour can be expected. Where blindness is temporary, ensure that the child is aware of this. It is important that the child should never be given a date on which to expect that his bandages will be removed or his sight return unless the staff are absolutely certain when this will be.

If blindness is permanent, a multidisciplinary approach towards obtaining expert help may be necessary, including, for example, a clinical psychologist, as psychological manifestations may continue to be present over a period of months or years.

The Effects of Monocular Vision

The parents, who may already be experiencing guilt feelings, may be very aware of the fact their child now "has only one eye" and may become over-protective to try to prevent the possibility of further injury. A child who is blind in one eye may be excluded from certain careers – e.g. pilot, heavy goods driver and any job that involves detailed fine movements, such as assembling electronic components, microsurgery or watch and clock repairs – as monocular vision may lead to lack of depth perception.

The Disfigured Eye

If an eye has extensive scarring of the cornea or has shrunk through loss of ocular tissue, it will look unsightly and may lead to further psychological problems for the child. In this instance the parents will need guidance regarding management. In cosmetic terms it may be better to remove the eye and have an artificial eye fitted, and this will also be the case if a blind eye becomes painful. The parents and child should be encouraged to visit the artificial eye department during the preoperative period so that they can observe how the eyes are made.

In Manchester it takes about four weeks for an eye to be made, as each one is moulded and hand-painted to suit individual requirements. This service, based at a regional centre, is not available everywhere; consequently, some children may be less fortunate in obtaining a perfect match. For the period prior to insertion of the artificial eye a temporary clear plastic shell may be provided to prevent the socket from shrinking.

Prevention of Ophthalmic Injuries

Government regulations, for example the enforcement of the wearing of seat belts in cars and laws controlling the sale of fireworks and firearms and other weapons, have been responsible for a reduction in the number of ophthalmic injuries. A shopkeeper wishing to sell fireworks must be registered with the local authority, and strict regulations apply to the storage of fireworks. Furthermore, it is an offence to sell fireworks to anyone who is or appears to be under 16 years old. Fire Brigade personnel are happy to visit schools and children's hospitals to inform children of the dangers of fireworks and to explain the Fireworks Code. Crombie (1982) reports how, over a 10-year period in Newcastle-upon-Tyne, better education backed by appropriate legislation has decreased the incidence of eye injuries due to misuse or mishandling of fireworks from 30 deaths per annum to none.

Airgun pellet injuries, which are usually severe, remain a cause for concern. It is illegal to carry a loaded air weapon in a public place, to shoot at a bird or animal, and to discharge an air weapon in the street or within 50 ft. of the centre of a highway. Children between the ages of 14 and 17 cannot buy or hire an air weapon, but they can receive an air rifle as a gift. Children under 14 may not be given, hire or otherwise own an air rifle. However, they may use an air rifle if supervised by a person over 21 years of age. It must be remembered that air weapons are not toys but potentially dangerous fire arms. Eye injuries from air pellets are still occurring at the rate of about 35 a year in Manchester.

Many household substances, such as bleach, washing-up liquid and aerosol sprays, could be labelled to include information about their effect as irritants on the eye. Manufacturers could also be encouraged to include first aid and eye irrigation instructions on their packaging.

Parents need to become aware of the dangers inherent in cheap imported toys or those bought while on holiday abroad. The manufacture of foreign toys is often not subject to strict safety standards: consequently, it has been known for many imported toys to have removable parts with sharp stalks and for clockwork toys to break easily, propelling small objects in different directions.

In eye injury prevention it is also important that potentially dangerous implements such as scissors, razor blades and knives be safely stored.

As the use of sunlamps becomes more popular the public needs to be better informed on the importance of wearing goggles while using them.

Summary

Crombie (1982) notes that more eyes are lost as the result of injury in the first decade of life than in any other. In absolute terms this means that in the UK 350 children's eyes per annum are lost following injury, i.e. approximately one eye every day of the year. The consequences for the children involved include those which have their basis in cosmetic problems, which can later manifest as serious psychological disturbances. Although lack of depth perception can usually be overcome by retraining the brain to appreciate depth with one eye rather than two, visual acuity is not always as good with one eye as it is with two. The result of this is that the child will always be excluded from certain occupations.

It has been demonstrated that eye injuries of any type can often result in continuing episodes of inflammation to the injured eye, resulting in pain, deterioration in vision and loss of schooling. Eye injuries of whatever sort, therefore, can affect a child for life.

Reference

Crombie A L (1982) Ocular injuries to children. *Safety Education*, Autumn: 12–13.

Recommended Reading

In Touch. A BBC publication on aids and services for blind and partially sighted people. London: BBC.
Royal National Institute for the Blind (1980) *Toys with a Purpose*. London: RNIB.
Royal National Institute for the Blind (1986) *Choices for Children: Educational Opportunities for Visually Handicapped Children and Young People*. London: RNIB.
Royal National Institute for the Blind (1989) *One Step at a Time*. London: RNIB.

Scott E P, Ian J E and Freeman R D (1985) *Can't Your Child See?* Baltimore: University Park Press.
Voluntary Council for Handicapped Children (1976) *Help Starts Here.* Booklet of welfare rights and helpful addresses. London: National Childrens Bureau.

Useful Addresses

Advisory Centre for Education
18 Victoria Park Square
London E2 9PB

National Childrens Bureau
8 Wakely Street
London EC1V 7QE

Parents Telephone Advisory Service
(Advice for parents of blind children)
Northampton (0604) 407726

Royal National Institute for the Blind (RNIB) and RNIB Education Advisory Service
224–6–8 Portland Street
London W1N 6AA

Toy Library Association
Seabrook House
Wyllyotts Manor
Darkes Lane
Potters Bar
Hertfordshire EN6 2HL

Chapter 9
Fractures, Sprains and Soft Tissue Injuries

Margaret Morgan   Donna Mead

Fractures, sprains and soft tissue injuries, particularly in children, are normally envisaged as the main workload of an Accident and Emergency Department. They account for 22 500 children being admitted to hospital in England and Wales in one year (CAPT, 1983) with approximately 2000 children each year losing an average of 30 days' schooling as a result of fractures needing hospital treatment.

Other sequelae include the immediate consequences of the injury for the child and his family. For the child, there is pain, distress, shock, anxiety, uncomfortable treatment and the effects of hospitalisation. For the family, it means being called away from work or home, possibly via police messages, hasty arrangements for the care of other siblings, getting to the hospital and great anxiety until the nature of the injury is discovered. Teachers may be involved if the injury happens at school, and may have to leave a class to accompany a child to hospital until the parents arrive. But when all this has calmed down, treatment has been given and all have returned home, it is the long-term consequences that will most affect the child and his family.

The treatments for fractures and sprains are designed to immobilise the injured limb(s) and advice given usually includes an initial period of bed rest. The child is, therefore, usually kept away from school, sometimes for long periods, which can have serious effects on his educational progress. If a period in hospital is necessary, the child will be subject to the effects of separation from family and friends. When the treatment is completed and plaster casts or strappings are removed, further problems can occur from continuing pain, muscle weakness or limb deformity. The child may not be prepared for this, feeling that once the plaster is removed he will be able to return to his normal behaviour. Wolff (1969) described children's feelings of disappointment when this was not so, and how children sometimes developed regressive behaviour, for example bedwetting or soiling. Limb deformity or shortening has an effect on the child's ability to take part in normal play and game activities. It may take some time for the child to adjust to his limited function and regain use of the limb. Younger children can usually cope with any deformity well, but the school age child will find adjustment more difficult, particularly if subjected to teasing and ridicule at school.

Causes of Fractures, Sprains and Soft Tissue Injuries

The majority of traumatic injuries are caused through normal play, either in the home (13 per cent of all fractures requiring hospital treatment in 1983), at school (0.2 per cent of fractures requiring admission) or in the community (road traffic accidents forming 10 per cent of admissions).

In the home parents can greatly influence the child's play environment to reduce the risk of injury. The parent's ability and willingness to create a safe environment can be enhanced by receiving appropriate prevention advice from the health-care professional. In terms of fractures, sprains and soft tissue injuries such advice could include the following:

1. Safety gates on stairs to prevent injury from falls.
2. Advice against changing the baby's nappy on high surfaces, for example kitchen table or work surface, as falls occur when the baby is left unattended.
3. Door jams to prevent doors slamming shut completely, thus reducing the chance of trapped finger injuries.
4. Tacking down loose carpets to prevent slipping and injury.
5. Regular maintenance and servicing of the child's play equipment, for example bicycles, roller skates, swings and slides, to reduce the risk of injury through faulty equipment.

At school there are the obvious risks of fractures, sprains and other injuries during gymnastics, competition sports and team games. The maintenance of sports equipment and supervision during sports activities is the responsibility of the teachers and school authorities. School summer camps or day trips also carry risks, and injuries can occur during walking and climbing expeditions.

It is difficult for any child supervisor to strike the correct balance between preventing unnecessary accidents and over-protecting the child, who is learning through play.

Outside the home and school, the child is at risk of injury in parks, in playgrounds and on the streets. Playground development in this country has followed the lead of other European countries. As outlined elsewhere in the book the main improvements have been:

1. high slides being set into banks of earth so that the falling distance is reduced;
2. areas under swings and climbing equipment being changed from hard cement or tarmac to softer bark chippings or rubber to reduce the impact of a fall;
3. swings now being made of rubber to reduce the force of impact if a child is hit.

Unauthorised playgrounds cause more of a problem. Building sites, unoccupied houses, rubbish dumps – any area, in fact, that is not regularly supervised –

all provide an exciting and different challenge to the child, and all are potentially dangerous. Decreasing the accessibility of these areas or increasing their supervision, through improved site security for example, and educating the child on the dangers of playing in such areas, are perhaps the only effective measures of accident prevention.

Road traffic accidents are a cause of multiple fractures and injuries to children. As mentioned elsewhere, children are frequently allowed onto roads or pavements unsupervised. Their perception of danger is different from that of adults, and, according to Wolff (1969), they are not always aware of the power of motorised vehicles. Road safety and information campaigns are aimed at improving the child's appreciation of the dangers involved.

Fractures

The bones of young children are supple and difficult to fracture completely. Injury usually results in greenstick fractures, so called because they resemble the damage caused to a young, green branch when bent. All fractures in children tend to heal more quickly than in adults and can eventually regain bone outline as the child grows, even if incomplete reduction of the fracture is achieved or overcalcification occurs. However, the fact that the child is still growing can cause problems if damage occurs to the epiphyses of the long bones. The child's growth then needs to be checked regularly by the orthopaedic specialist.

Compound fractures of the radius, ulna and lower limbs are caused by violent injury and are becoming more common with the use of high speed (BMX) bikes, and skateboards and through road traffic accidents. Comminuted fractures are rare in children.

With any fracture or injury, particularly in a young child, the possibility of non-accidental injury should be considered and if suspicion is aroused, carefully investigated.

The principal fractures that occur in children, their cause and main points of treatment, are outlined in Appendix I of this chapter.

Sprains

Injury during normal boisterous play or through accidents does not always result in fractures. Sprained muscles surrounding a joint, with resultant bleeding into the tissues, can give rise to as much, if not more, swelling and pain as a fracture. After examination by the doctor and check X-rays, if necessary, have discounted the possibility of a fracture, treatment is usually that of supporting the joint with either a padded crêpe bandage if swelling is severe, or Elastoplast strapping, tubigrip or even a plaster of Paris cast.

Exact application techniques will vary from hospital to hospital, but the principles of applying a bandage are:

1. to apply the crêpe bandage over the top of a single layer of gamgee, firmly, but not tightly, to allow for further swelling;
2. that the padded bandage should extend well above and below the affected joint;

3. to avoid excessive movement of the joint when applying the bandage: the joint should not be forced into the correct position if it is very painful to do so or it is swollen;

4. that time spent getting the trust of parents and child and gentle handling and care when giving treatment will make return visits less stressful for everyone.

The principles of applying an Elastoplast strapping are:

1. it is kinder to put a length of close fitting stockinette under the Elastoplast strapping, leaving a gap at the top and bottom of the bandage for the Elastoplast to stick to the limb; removal is then less traumatic but the bandage should still remain in place;

2. again, the Elastoplast should not be stretched onto the limb, but laid on to avoid constriction; for the same reason, it should not be applied in a figure of eight arrangement around a joint;

The Elastoplast is usually left in place for 10–14 days and resting the limb is advised. Children in the youngest age group (nought to four years old) may find a way of removing or loosening the strapping before their next appointment, and parents should be advised to return to the hospital or surgery if the strapping becomes too loose to be effective.

Return is also advised if the limb above and below the bandage becomes cold or discoloured, indicating blood flow impairment, if the child complains of increasing pain, which could indicate a more serious injury, or if the sprain does not resolve after the initial treatment, at which point immobilisation in a plaster cast may be considered.

Younger children cannot reasonably be restrained and watched continuously and will often try to continue their normal activities despite the injury. Suitable age-appropriate play activities are outlined at the end of this chapter. School-age children will also want to return to normal play and, again, restriction of activity is difficult for the parents to impose. Thus, reasonable guidelines must be given and achievable goals set, or they are more likely than not to be ignored.

Parents should not be made to feel guilty if they return with the child before the stated date with the bandage completely or partially removed. It can easily be re-applied, and although this may take up time, it will achieve a better end result for that child. Parents may well try to find other and perhaps inappropriate treatments, or avoid returning, if they feel that the nurse or doctor will disapprove of their early return.

As with all advice, information must be clear and be given both verbally and in writing.

Plaster of Paris Casts – Application and Nursing Care

As outlined in Appendix I of this chapter, the immobilisation of the fracture, usually including the joint above and below it, is most commonly achieved through the application of a Plaster of Paris (POP) cast or the more expensive, but lightweight, waterproof cast.

The application requires skill and a supply of POP or resin bandages, as well as the back-up of orthopaedic and X-ray facilities. POP and resin casts are usually applied in the Accident and Emergency Department in an area away from the normal dressing area that is specifically designated for the purpose, as the process is messy and requires space. As with all treatment areas used by children, bright walls and ceiling, posters and a supply of toys for distraction are essential.

The older child will be receptive to explanations of the procedure and, unless very confused or frightened, will co-operate while the cast is being applied. If there are no other complications, such as head injury, Entonox gas or an analgesic can be considered if applying the cast will be painful. Even with the older child it takes two people to apply a cast satisfactorily as it is not easy for the patient to support his own injured arm for any length of time.

The exact method of application of a POP or resin cast will not be explained in detail as every hospital has its own policy, but general points for application include:

1. Application should be carried out as quickly and as smoothly as possible to avoid movement of the fracture and unnecessary pain.
2. The X-ray of the affected limb should be referred to prior to application to ensure that the cast is correct for the type of fracture and is applied to the correct limb. The X-ray can also be used to re-explain the injury and treatment to the parents and child.
3. The fracture site should be adequately supported throughout the procedure to prevent excess movement.

Application is commenced around the fracture site to give support to the fracture.

General Approaches to Applying POP Casts

Birth to 3 years old   Verbal explanation of the procedure may only exacerbate the child's fear and will not be well understood, but the parents usually need a full explanation to allay their fears. A demonstration using a small strip of POP and the child's doll or teddy bear, or even a brother or sister's finger, will be of greater use than just a verbal explanation in preparing the child.

If the parents are willing, it is often easier and kinder not to separate the child from them. The child can sit on his mother or father's well-protected lap, with one nurse standing either behind the parent to support an arm or in front to support a leg.

Constant talk by the nurse applying the cast will help to calm the child; simple explanations, such as when you are going to apply the stockinette sock or glove (if used) and telling the child to listen for the bubbles when the plaster roll is put into the water, may be of benefit. Soft toys, mobiles or activity centres can help to distract attention. However, there are some situations in which the child will not be pacified or distressed, and it is better just to get on with the application as speedily as possible.

It is important to explain that the POP cast will get warm, but not too hot, after application, which will help to ease the pain, and that it will go cold as it sets hard.

3–6 Years old   This age group will respond to simple explanations beforehand but, again, demonstration is very helpful. As before, it is better if the child can sit on his mother or father's lap during application of the cast, and constant explanation at every stage will help to settle fears and apprehension.

Yet again, time spent before application in getting the child in the right psychological state can save a lot of time during application when, hopefully, the child will be co-operative.

6–12 Years old   Explanation of the procedure is usually taken well. Parents and child can be given some simple explanations and shown the X-rays prior to application of the POP. The child is usually happy to sit or lie down on his own, with his parents watching.

Being positive about the cast, such as stressing that it can be written and drawn on when dry, will help the child look forward to the application instead of seeing it as a threat.

Girls of this age can already be very conscious of their appearance, but some positive images can usually be found, for example, using their mother's scarf as a sling or buying a new one, or showing them interesting and fun ways of wearing their clothes around the cast.

Following Application of POP

Immediately following application, the POP cast will still be soft and should be handled with the palms of the hands, not the fingers, because these can cause ridges in the plaster and lead to sores of the skin underneath. The limb should be supported by soft pillows or in a sling.

Parents, and child if old enough, should be given both oral and written instructions on the care of the POP cast, which should include:

1.   the importance of careful handling until the cast is fully dry;
2.   no weight bearing on a leg POP until a walking sole has been applied;
3.   no writing on the POP until it is dry, as this can cause indentation leading to skin sores;
4.   finger or toe exercises to reduce swelling and to maintain muscle tone;
5.   that parents should return with the child if his fingers (or toes) become cold or blue, indicating circulatory impairment;
6.   that a return is also needed if the POP becomes wet and therefore ineffective;
7.   that sharp objects, such as knitting needles, should not be inserted into the plaster to relieve itching as this damages the skin and can cause sores.

Most children return to be seen by the orthopaedic specialist the day after injury so that the treatment given and the child's condition can be checked. Subsequent appointments are given at this time.

Instructions for care can again be given or re-inforced, and advice on returning to school or regular activities will be useful for the parents now that the initial panic has gone.

Hospitalisation

The child is usually admitted to hospital for observation in the following situations:

1. Displaced fractures that have been difficult to manipulate, where swelling is likely to occur around the fracture site and compromise the circulation.
2. Fractures of the elbow, particularly supracondylar fractures, where manipulation has been necessary and excessive swelling may occur.
3. Following accidents where other injuries, particularly head and suspected internal injuries, have been sustained.
4. Compound fractures, which need manipulation, and often internal fixation, in a sterile theatre.
5. Fractures that cannot be immobilised using a POP or resin cast, where long-term hospitalisation and fixed traction are needed.

As outlined in Appendix I, the main fractures requiring traction are:

1. fractures of the femur, where a Thomas splint is used for older children and gallows traction for younger children;
2. severe compound or comminuted fractures that have required internal fixation.

Long-term hospitalisation may also be necessary if multiple fractures involving more than one limb, e.g. fractures of both arms in a child who has fallen out of a tree, have occurred.

It can be seen that the hospitalised child with a fracture may be either fairly mobile with only a POP cast or immobilised with traction or because of multiple injuries. A wide range of nursing care is, therefore, required for these children. The main nursing approaches are described below.

Care of the Immobilised Child in Traction

In the initial period following admission, the child will not want to move and will still be recovering from the physical effects of the accident. During this time particular attention needs to be paid to maintaining skin integrity. The main aspects of nursing care of the immobilised child are outlined in Appendix II of this chapter, with specific care of the child with a Thomas splint in Appendix III. However, once the child has recovered and any pain has subsided, he will be able and willing to move around the bed. Much of this initial care, which of necessity focuses on physical needs, can now be directed towards the more psychological and social problems of the child. These can be broadly split into four main areas:

1. Boredom.
2. Separation from family and friends.

3. Loss of independence.
4. Interrupted schooling.

Boredom This is a big problem, common to all age groups. The loss of mobility and the possible loss of use of either arms or legs means that normal methods of play may not be possible. Imaginative play methods, adapted according to the child's age, can help to occupy his mind and assist in rehabilitation if fairly long-term loss of use of limbs is faced: for example, a child with a fractured upper end of tibia, who may have been hospitalised initially and who then goes home with a full-length plaster, which will be in place for six weeks, needs to be taught different ways of getting around and playing. Assessing and planning the child's needs will require a multidisciplinary team approach, with input from nursing, medical, occupational therapy, hospital, school and physiotherapy staff and the family. If age and circumstances allow, the child should be involved in such planning. A plan of care can then be drawn up, with each team member using his particular expertise. Some suggestions for each age group are outlined below.

Birth to 4 Years old.
Leg immobilised:

1. As with adults, a simple bar or handle can be suspended above the child (when of appropriate age) to help him pull himself up.
2. An angled mirror, also suspended above him, will help the child to see what is going on, eat and watch television.
3. Mobiles or pictures above the bed give the child something to look at.
4. An angled, adjustable board mounted on a base to fit across the bed will enable the child to draw, paint and read while lying flat.
5. Toe-puppets, using the characters with rhymes, will make exercise more fun.

Arm immobilised:

1. Even if he normally writes or draws with the immobilised hand, a small child will quickly adapt to using the opposite arm.
2. Toys that require fine manipulation or which have difficult catches should be avoided.
3. Finger-puppets will encourage finger exercise.
4. Toys, drinks, food, books, etc. should be placed within reach of the child's undamaged arm.
5. Bean bags can be used to prop the child upright.

5–12 Years old.

1. Mirrors, pictures, a lifting handle and angled bed board can be used, as above.
2. Tape-cassette programmes, which have books to go with them, will both sustain interest and help the child's reading.
3. Stories read to the children about other children in hospital and in plaster will help them to verbalise their own feelings. These include:

Going to Hospital, by Althea (1974), published by Dinosaur Publications, London

A Crocodile Plaster, by Marjorie-Ann Watts (1978), published by André Deutsch, London

Simon Goes to Hospital, a comic available from NAWCH, London

4. Creative play ideas include:

- Drawing.
- Finger painting.
- Potato prints.
- Glueing and cutting.
- Modelling – clay, Playdough, Plasticine, plaster of Paris.
- Threading – macaroni, buttons, straw, paper, beads, anything with holes in.
- Musical activities – if all the children are moved into one bay (preferably with a door!) they can sing, bang trays, tins and cups, shake containers filled with beads, rice, etc., strike tambourines, triangles and bells, and use their hands and arms to 'dance' with the music.

Separation from Family and Friends A lengthy stay in hospital affects relations within the family. During the initial traumatic period, one or both parents will usually stay with the child in hospital. The treatment of serious fractures, however, is prolonged, requiring an average stay of 31 days in hospital. This attention, therefore, cannot usually be sustained, and separation of the child from the family is inevitable. Some parents will want to spend the majority of their time with the child and this can cause friction and tension between partners if home life is neglected. It is important that the parents understand that it is important to set time aside for themselves during this period without feeling guilty. It is also important that the child is able to form attachments with the nurses who will care for him during his parents' absence. In keeping with current recommendations, therefore, it is essential that the child receives care from his allocated nurse wherever possible, thus avoiding the problems that may arise when there are many care givers.

Whenever possible, however, family involvement in the delivery of care is recommended to help to overcome the effects of separation. Depending on the child's age, contact with family and friends may be maintained by letter and by taped messages from classmates; pictures of family members, pets or friends, for example a class, Brownie or Cub pack photograph, can be displayed as the child wishes. This problem is discussed in more detail in Chapter 4.

Loss of Independence As a result of the treatment necessary for his injuries, the child may face a period during which any independence previously gained, for example, using a spoon or fork to feed himself, or using the toilet instead of the potty, may be curtailed. Children may be very reluctant to give up these skills, and when forced to do so because of their injuries, they can become very frustrated. This may manifest itself by behaviour such as restlessness, irritability or aggression. This is a difficult problem because, as Wolff (1969) notes, if the effects of separation and loss of independence are severe, it is often difficult to distinguish the effects of being separated from the family from the effects of treatment. Adolescents, especially, resent any loss of independence. Their particular problems are discussed in detail in Chapter 4.

With creativity and patience some independence can be preserved, even for the toddler. In the case of adolescents, allowing them to make decisions about aspects of their care will lessen the undesirable effects of loss of independence, while at the same time allow them to participate in their own care whenever possible. The younger child, too, will react positively to being allowed to make decisions in relation to aspects of daily living activities, e.g. choosing meals or clothes.

Interrupted Schooling　The effects of this are also discussed in Chapter 4. Interrupted schooling is a difficult problem in the school-age child who requires long-term hospitalisation. Initially, because of the injuries and their treatment, educational activities are not appropriate. As treatment progresses and the child feels well, they should be re-introduced. Most paediatric wards with long-stay patients have organised hospital schools with teachers who work with the children to maintain their school-work. This is obviously most important for the secondary school age group, who may find difficulty in catching up with missed school work when they return to school, the child who may be approaching examinations may be particularly disadvantaged. For such children, it is essential that it is made possible for them to continue with their studies.

It can be seen that there is a wide range of fractures and sprains that can occur as a result of accidents in an equally wide range of situations. Clearly, it is not possible or desirable that all such accidents should be prevented. Fractures and sprains often occur as the result of normal, boisterous play and, as such, are very difficult to prevent. The role of the nursing profession is to support and encourage the family in their efforts to reduce the risks of accidents, and to help them to cope with the effects of the injuries when an accident has occurred.

Appendix I　Common Fractures, Causes and Treatment

Fracture location	Cause	Treatment
Lower Limb		
Phalanges	Stubbing toe. Bike trapping toe underneath pedal	Garter strapping metatarsal bar, padded bandage, Collodian splint – at the discretion of the doctor. Weighbearing allowed. No pressure on toes.

Appendix I, continued

Fracture location	Cause	Treatment

Metatarsals	Direct blow resulting in a crushing injury. Trapping of foot in a bicycle wheel. Sports injuries, e.g.:
	  Football: kick from opponent's foot
	  Hockey: from ball or stick.
	  Weight lifting: dropping equipment onto foot
		Below-knee POP. Non-weight-bearing. Crutches used
		  or
		Weight bearing allowed if tyre used.
		N.B. ensure that POP is dry 48 hours after application.

Ankle		
Fractured malleolus Bimalleolar (Pott's) fracture	Trapping of foot, which is violently rotated, either externally or internally; or vertical compression, i.e. landing on feet	Below-knee POP. Non-weight-bearing. Crutches used. Full-leg POP in children under four years of age
Pott's fracture with dislocation	As above.	Manipulation under anaesthetic. Below-knee POP. Non-weight-bearing. Crutches used. Full-leg POP if under four years of age
Fibula	Rarely occurs on its own. Usually associated with fractured tibia.	Full-leg POP if associated with fractured tibia. Non-weight-bearing for 48 hours until plaster dries. Then weight bearing allowed.
Tibia	Direct blow, e.g. road traffic accident in which the child is a pedestrian. Indirect violence of a twisting force e.g. falling from bicycle with foot caught in the wheel.	Generally full-length POP. Non-weight-bearing. Crutches used. When the lower third of the tibia is fractured, below-knee POP may be applied. Full-leg POP in children under four years of age
Knee		
Displaced patellar fracture	Sideways fall. Twisting games	Admission to hospital necessary. Manipulation under anaesthetic will probably be needed

Appendix I, continued

Fracture location	Cause	Treatment
Dislocated patellar fracture	Twisting knee, e.g. playing football	Robert Jones bandage applied initially. Later long-leg POP cylinder cast may be applied
Undisplaced fracture of patella	Fall straight onto knee.	As for dislocation of patellar. No manipulation under general anaesthetic.
		For all fractures of patellar: Initially non-weight-bearing. Following a period of rest, gradual increase to weight bearing
Femur (shaft)	Very hard blow involving direct violence. Road traffic accident or falls. Non-accidental injury	Infants: Gallows traction Other children: fixed traction on a Thomas splint. Bed rest, non-weight-bearing
Upper Limb		
Thumb	Direct violence. Being hit with a heavy object	Immobilisation with, for example: 1. thumb spica cast 2. Bennett's POP 3. Zimmer splint if fracture is distal
First metacarpal (Bennett's fracture)	Fist fight	As for fractured thumb
Scaphoid	Fall onto out-stretched hand, thumb bent back	Scaphoid plaster cast. Fracture may not show up on X-ray until two weeks after injury
Fifth metacarpal	Direct violence, e.g. fist fight or hitting any solid object, e.g. a wall	Extended Colle's plaster cast
Phalanges	Fall onto hand. Hit by a solid object	Distal: Immobilised in a mallet or Zimmer plaster Medial: Two-finger strapping Proximal: Zimmer splint If fracture is displaced, manipulation under anaesthetic may be necessary

Appendix I, continued

Fracture location	Cause	Treatment
Forearm		
Radius greenstick fracture	Fall occurring in a young child	1. Below-elbow POP 2. Below-elbow back slab 3. Full-arm POP in very small, active child
Shaft of radius/ulna	Falls	If fracture is undisplaced, above-elbow POP. If fracture is displaced, manipulation under anaesthetic and above-elbow POP
Head of radius	Direct violence to elbow, or external or internal rotation	If undisplaced, immobilise in collar and cuff/sling. If displaced, general anaesthetic necessary for evulsion of head of radius; immobilise in collar and cuff/sling
Supracondylar fracture	Backward fall or blow	If undisplaced, collar and cuff sling. If displaced, manipulation under anaesthetic necessary. Child admitted so that pulses can be checked
Shaft of humerus	Direct blow. Force transferred to upper arm following a fall onto an outstretched arm	Immobilisation in either: 1. collar and cuff 2. gutter splint 3. U-slab
Neck of humerus	Fall onto shoulder, e.g. rugby tackle	If undisplaced, collar and cuff. If displaced, manipulation under anaesthetic, then collar and cuff
Scapula	Direct blow	Sling
Clavicle	Fall with out-stretched hand onto shoulder	Figure-of-eight bandage. Collar and cuff or sling on arm of affected side

Appendix II   General Nursing Care of the Immobilized Child in Bed

Problem	Nursing action	Rationale
Potential problems of skin breakdown due to enforced immobility	Change position of child four-hourly or as frequently as necessary.	Relieves pressure on pressure points. If easing to either side is not possible, rubber rings, sheepskin pads, pillow or orthopaedic foam can help cushion pressure points
	Gentle massage of pressure points, particularly buttocks, shoulders, heels, four-hourly	Increases blood supply to area to help prevent ischaemic damage sores
	Do not rub	Force and excessive movement of skin may cause further damage
	Observe and record child's general condition: to include changes in sensation, skin irritation, pain, attitude	Changes in sensation, particularly pain, can indicate possible problems and should be investigated. For example, heat and pain in isolated area (particularly under POP) could indicate developing pressure sore, irritation under plaster extensions could be response to adhesive or bandage, lethargy or irritability could be infection
Boredom	Imaginative use of games and play. Provide resources for play and relaxation. Devise specific plan of activities with multidisciplinary team	See text

Appendix II, continued

Problem	Nursing action	Rationale
Separation from family and friends	Encourage family to participate in all aspects of implementing care. Involve family in care planning. Encourage and facilitate visiting by offering unrestricted visiting times, financial help with fares, information and crêche/nursery for other siblings, and support groups. Offer support to child in lieu of parents when parents unable to visit. Promote ward atmosphere conducive to family centred care	See text, also Chapter 4
Loss of independence	Allow and encourage child to participate in maximum amount of self-care. Retrain where necessary. Maintain child's dignity when carrying out nursing care	To allow and promote independence in those areas of his care not affected by the treatment/injuries
	Promote personalised care where possible, i.e. allow child to keep own belongings, routine and diet	To keep changes to a minimum; child will have own things as 'anchor' and be able to adjust to unavoidable changes such as loss of independence
Interrupted schooling	Provide facilities, materials and routine to encourage maintenance of learning	See text
	Plan daily routine to include school work	
	Facilitate and help hospital school teachers to maintain learning	

Appendix III   Nursing Care for the Child with Skin Traction (Thomas Splint) – Specific Care Related to the Splint

Thomas splint traction uses a frame (the splint) to provide an anchor for skin traction in order to immobilize the whole limb. The tapes secured to the distal W-shaped end of the splint exert traction, while counter-traction is exerted by the pressure of the padded ring on the prominent ischial tuberosity.

Potential problem	Nursing action	Rationale
Interference with circulation to limb by swelling and/or pressure of equipment.	Check gap between ring and skin as required; immediately on admission, then two-hourly, four-hourly when swelling subsides	Haemorrhage and oedema around the fracture site (femur) cause swelling. Previously loose rings may then be too tight; these cannot expand and may need to be changed
	Observe and report changes in limb, colour, sensation and temperature	
Skin breakdown due to continuous contact with equipment and bed linen	Check skin under bandages for blisters, sores and dryness four-hourly. In particular inspect groin for signs of soreness	Some children develop blisters under extension plates in reaction to adhesive. Crêpe bandages can dry the skin. Wrinkles in bandages can cause sores.
		Early detection and treatment of pressure sores prevents further skin damage and pain
	Ensure leather and padding of ring is in good repair. Rub olive oil into leather if necessary to keep it supple	Cracked leather can cause damage to skin, particularly over pressure points. Inadequate padding will not provide protection from pressure of a hard metal splint
	Gently ease skin underneath the ring of the splint every four hours and more frequently if there are signs of pressure or damage	Releasing pressure of ring on one area of the skin reduces risk of pressure sores
	Gently massage skin underneath the splint. Do not rub	Force and excessive movement of skin may cause further skin damage

Appendix III, continued

Potential problem	Nursing action	Rationale
	If appropriate, ensure child changes position frequently; use monkey bar if appropriate. Position of heels should be changed as part of active leg exercises. Sheepskin heel muffs may be used.	To prevent sores on immobilised heel caused by pressure from bed. Heel muff provides softer resting point
Lost muscle tone	Calf and thigh: Encourage child to carry out active exercise by plantar flexing and dorsiflexing foot, and tensing calf at least every four hours. Use passive exercises in unconscious or severely injured child	To prevent muscle wasting during period of inactivity. Recovery of full function when mobilisation commences will be impaired if muscle tone is poor
	Patella: Thigh exercises will also mobilise patella. Check patellar movement every four hours	
Hip contractures due to prolonged immobilisation in one position	Ensure that child alternates position from semi-recumbent to lying flat approx. three-hourly	Prevents hip contractures occurring as a result of enforced immobility
Effective traction not maintained due to loss of alignment or malalignment of traction	Check adhesion of skin extension plasters 4-hourly	Extension plasters form fixed point for traction. If loose, traction is not effective
	Check four-hourly that weights used on traction are running through pulleys and are hanging freely	If weights are restricted, traction will be variable or reduced
	Make sure that counter-traction is provided. Foot of child's bed may have to be raised to counteract traction weight and prevent child being pulled to end of bed	Child's weight is often insufficient to provide counter-traction

Reference

Wolff S (1969) *Children Under Stress*. London: Trend and Co.

Recommended Reading

Child Accident Prevention Trust (1983) *Hospital In-patient Enquiry*. London: CAPT.

Freud A (1946) *The Ego and the Mechanisms of Defence*. London: Hogarth Press.

Freud A (1952) *The Role of Bodily Illness in the Mental Life of Children*. London: Hogarth Press.

Greenwood A (1984) *Your Child in an Immobilising Plaster*. London: NAWCH.

Illingworth C (1982) *The Diagnosis and Primary Care of Accidents and Emergencies in Children*. Oxford: Blackwell Scientific.

Klein M (1964) The psychoanalytic play technnique. In: *Child Psychotherapy* ed. Howarth M R pp. 119–120. London: Basic Books.

Levey H, Sheldon S and Rabi S (1984) *Diagnosis and Management of the Hospitalized Child*. New York: Raven Press.

Prugh D G (1953) A study of the emotional reactions of children and families to hospitalization and illness. *American Journal of Ortho-psychiatry*, **23**: 70.

Chapter 10
Thermal Injuries
Anna Foreshaw   Eileen Bottomly

Despite considerable publicity, the incidence of thermal injury remains high. In England and Wales in 1985, 119 children between 0 and 14 years of age died from fire, flames, burns and scalds, most of these as a result of inhalation of smoke and toxic fumes. Many of the cases came from deprived families with multiple problems. The Child Accident Prevention Trust reports that between 2500 and 3000 children are admitted to hospital as a result of scalds, with a similar number for burns, each year in England and Wales. In addition, approximately 30 000 children in England and Wales attend hospital each year due to scalds with 20 000 children attending hospital as a result of burns (CAPT, 1987a,b). Long-term sequelae, such as psychological trauma and scars, can affect children's lives dramatically for many years. The three interlinked factors involved in domestic accidents, As examined by Gaffin (1981), are:

1. the child;
2. the cause of injury;
3. the environment.

The Child

Children have different types of thermal injury at different ages, relating to their stage of development.

Birth to 1 Year Old

Scalds are by far the most common injury in this age group. As the child's motor skills are not fully developed, he is not totally mobile, and if containers of hot liquid are accessible, he is likely to grasp them for support, tipping the fluid over himself.

1–5 Years Old

These years are a new and exciting phase in a child's life. He is now developing new skills such as mobility and will, therefore, explore his surroundings. Unfortunately, he is at greater risk of scalding because he is totally unaware of danger. Objects such as pans, bottles, teapots, cups of tea and baths – which are all items in a normal household containing hot liquids – can prove lethal to children of this age group.

5–10 Years Old

The child is now starting school and gaining more independence. He is becoming more inquisitive, and reduced parental supervision means that he is likely to become more mischievous. Children of this age group spend more time in pursuit of outdoor activities. Being adventurous, they are at a higher risk of thermal injuries, for example those caused as a result of playing with matches or fires.

10–16 Years Old

In keeping with the trend in the pattern of accidents sustained by adolescents, more boys than girls sustain thermal injuries. The activities of children of this age group are mainly outdoor, and boys are at high risk for burns as they experiment with fire, petrol, railway lines and electricity pylons. Children in this age group are likely to sustain serious injuries, particularly to hands, face and legs.

   The professional who encounters a child who has sustained a thermal injury should always consider the possibility of non-accidental injury, particularly in children from birth to three years of age. An unusual pattern of distribution of the injury may indicate the need to make such a differentiation.

The Cause of Injury

Figure 10.1 shows the common causes of thermal injuries. The agent responsible is related to the child's stage of development.

The Environment

The majority of children who sustain thermal injuries come from families in the lower income group living in overcrowded conditions with poor facilities. Often these are large or one-parent families, which places the parent under great stress and supervision of the child tends to be intermittent. While environment alone cannot cause thermal injury, it is a predisposing factor to accidents.

Classification of Injury

Injuries caused by burns and scalds are classified according to the depth of tissue destroyed. For the injuries to heal within the specified time periods, the wound must not become contaminated with microorganisms, as infection causes further loss of tissue, which lengthens the time required for healing and increases the incidence of scar tissue formation.

Superficial Injury

While this type of injury mainly results in the destruction of the epidermis, a small section of the dermis may be involved. The wound should heal within

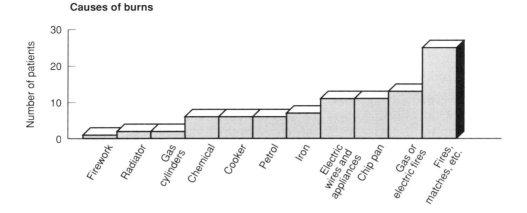

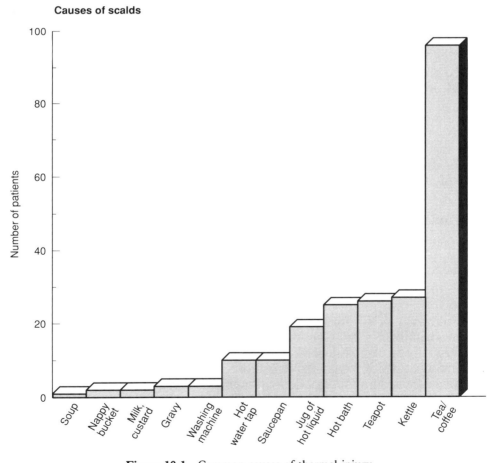

Figure 10.1 Common causes of thermal injury

10–14 days and will not produce any permanent disfigurement after the capillaries have closed and the extra blood supply has been diverted from the area.

Partial-thickness Injury

Partial-thickness injury causes destruction of the epidermis and approximately half the dermis; healing takes place from the remaining epithelialising elements of the dermis. This type of wound should heal within 14–21 days and should not produce permanent disfigurement.

Deep Dermal Injury

Deep dermal injuries result from the destruction of the epidermis and most of the dermis, leaving only a small proportion of elements from which epithelialisation can take place. The wound will take at least 21–28 days to heal, but will invariably require a skin graft to provide adequate skin cover. This injury will produce some permanent disfigurement.

Full-thickness Injury

Full-thickness injury leads to total destruction of the epidermis and dermis, and may extend to the subcutaneous fat, muscle and bone. All such injuries require a skin graft to provide skin cover, and gross disfigurement is inevitable.

Care of the Child with Minor Thermal Injuries

A burns dressing and after-care clinic, with clinical expertise, reduces the need for hospitalisation for most children who have sustained a minor thermal injury.

Superficial Injury

Following assessment of the extent of the injury, the gaseous analgesic agent Entonox is administered if required. Entonox is a mixture of 50% nitrous oxide and 50% oxygen, which provides a safe and easy method of pain relief and may obviate the need for a general anaesthetic or the administration of drugs by injection.

Debridement of all blisters and debris, using an antiseptic solution such as 0.05% cetrimide solution is carried out. The wound may be dressed with paraffin gauze, gauze soaked in a solution of 0.05% aqueous Hibitaine, or dry gauze secured by a crêpe bandage; this provides a pressure dressing that encourages the healing process. The dressing should remain intact for a further five days, after which the wound should be healed, unless there has been contamination with microorganisms.

Partial-thickness Injury

This type of injury is treated in the same way as a superficial injury for the first five to seven days. As there may be small areas of deep dermal destruction, the second dressing may require the application of an appropriate desloughing agent to aid separation of debris and promote wound healing. If the wound shows evidence of infection, swabs should be taken for culture and sensitivity (before an appropriate antiseptic is applied topically) and systemic antibiotics prescribed.

The parents must be reassured and given advice regarding care of the child at home, and should be encouraged to contact staff if any problems occur.

Care of the Child with Major Thermal Injuries

Any thermal injury that constitutes over 10 per cent destruction of the body surface is classified as major. Many of these injuries are full thickness and will require skin grafts. Where feasible, children with major burn injuries should be admitted direct to the burns unit.

The child's parents are likely to be shocked and distressed because of the sudden impact of the accident, and for this reason it is normal to obtain the initial history of the accident from the ambulance staff.

In keeping with the care required for any injured child, a child with severe thermal injuries will need a nursing approach that considers the physical, social and psychological needs of the child and family. This account of nursing care and management is divided into the needs of the child and family during the acute phase and post-shock period.

The Acute Phase

As soon as possible after admission, the child is attached to a monitor that records the core and skin temperatures, heart rate, blood pressure and respiration rate. Oxygen is administered to the child if there is a history of smoke inhalation or if respiratory distress is present.

The depth and percentage area of the injury is assessed using the Lund and Bower chart (Figure 10.2). Sedation such as morphine 0.2 mg/kg body weight may be administered on admission, and repeated six-hourly if required to alleviate the child's distress. Clothing is removed before the child's weight is determined.

The following investigations are performed on admission and as frequently as the child's condition necessitates throughout the shock period:

1. Packed cell volume.
2. Haemoglobin level.
3. Urea and electrolytes.
4. Blood gases.
5. Grouping and cross matching of blood.

Hypovolaemic Shock Hypovolaemic shock develops rapidly in major injuries because the heat at the time of injury causes vasodilation and an increased

Name: _____ Age: _____ Unit No: _____

Date of Observation: _____ Total % burn _____

% deep dermal _____

% full thickness _____

RELATIVE PERCENTAGE OF AREAS AFFECTED BY GROWTH

AREA	Age					
	0	1	5	10	15	Adult
A = $1/2$ of head	$9^{1}/_2$	$8^{1}/_2$	$6^{1}/_2$	$5^{1}/_2$	$4^{1}/_2$	$3^{1}/_2$
B = $1/2$ of one thigh	$2^{3}/_4$	$3^{1}/_4$	4	$4^{1}/_2$	$4^{1}/_2$	$4^{3}/_4$
C = $1/2$ of one leg	$2^{1}/_2$	$2^{1}/_2$	$2^{3}/_4$	3	$3^{1}/_4$	$3^{1}/_2$

Figure 10.2 Burns record

permeability, which results in circulatory fluid loss with subsequent haemocon-centration. The dehydration caused by excessive loss of fluid through burned tissue is a potentially serious problem, and the nursing actions taken to prevent and monitor this condition include:

1. insertion of an indwelling catheter so that urine output can be measured and urinalysis performed as often as necessary. Initially, oligurea will be present but as haemoconcentration is corrected a diuresis should occur. The urinary output during this period is a guide to renal function;
2. administration of plasma and intravenous fluids to replace the fluid lost. The volume of plasma required is calculated using the Muir and Barclay (1962) formula:

$$\frac{\text{Weight in kilograms} \times \text{percentage area of burn}}{2} = \text{No. of ml given in each period}$$
(see Table 10.1)

This quantity is given in each period for the first 36 hours, after which the capillaries begin to retain their tone.

Table 10.1   Definition of time periods for fluid replacement

Period	Time from injury, in hours
1	0–4
2	5–8
3	9–12
4	13–18
5	19–24
6	25–36

The child is also assessed clinically after each time period and the transfusion requirements adjusted accordingly. Maintenance fluids, such as 5 per cent dextrose and 0.45 per cent sodium chloride, are also required. Sodium chloride is necessary because the serum sodium will be low during the resuscitation phase. The volume of maintenance fluids is calculated according to the weight of the child:

<10 kg – 100 ml/kg per 24 hours
10–20 kg – 1000 ml + 50 ml/kg per 24 hours
>20 kg – 1500ml + 25 ml/kg per 24 hours

If the child becomes pyrexial, the maintenance fluids are increased by 10 per cent per 1°C rise in temperature. Once the haemoconcentration has been corrected, a low haemoglobin may be revealed, which may need to be restored with a blood transfusion.

After intravenous therapy has been commenced the wound is debrided and all blisters and debris are removed. The wound may be dressed with paraffin gauze soaked in an iodine-based disinfectant, such as Videne, or dry gauze to absorb serum, which is secured by a crêpe bandage.

Escharotomy   The tissue destroyed in a full-thickness injury becomes dry and unelastic and is termed the eschar. Areas of circumferential, full-thickness burns must be observed closely as the eschar acts as a tourniquet that will inhibit circulation to the limbs, or cause respiratory distress if the chest is affected. The circulation to the affected limb must be observed carefully to establish whether or not the blood supply is adequate: if it is, the limb will be pink and warm.

Escharotomy (cutting the eschar) will be performed if there are signs of a deterioration in the circulation. A longitudinal incision is made along the outer and inner aspect of the limb: this releases the tension and the circulation improves rapidly. The area is dressed with Videne to prevent infection.

Respiratory distress, which may be the result of inhalation injury, obstructive oedema or a tight eschar, is a potential problem. The nursing actions taken to prevent and monitor this condition include:

1.   careful examination of the nose and throat for soot and burned mucosa;
2.   observing the pattern of respiration closely for signs of distress. The child's position should be changed frequently and he should be encouraged to breathe deeply and cough. It may be necessary to hyperextend the neck to assist breathing;
3.   giving oxygen.

Hypothermia   Hypothermia may occur owing to excessive evaporation of tissue fluid or to exposure when the child is nursed exposed to the air. To prevent this problem the following nursing actions should be taken:

1.   Maintain the room temperature between 26°C and 33°C. The atmosphere should be humid.
2.   Provide a bed cradle with cover to prevent chilling.
3.   Avoid drafts.

Haemorrhage   Haemorrhage may result from injuries at the time of the accident or from erosion of blood vessels by debridement. The objective should be the early detection of bleeding, and nursing care therefore involves:

1.   elevating burned extremities, if possible;
2.   careful monitoring of the child's vital signs;
3.   avoiding the practice of reinforcing dressings as this could mask fresh bleeding;
4.   if fresh bleeding does occur, seeking emergency medical help.

During the resuscitation phase the parents may wish to stay with their child, and this should be encouraged. The parents will need constant reassurance at this time, which is given by ensuring that they are kept informed of all decisions concerning the child's management and that, where possible, they are involved in their child's care. Encouragement to eat and rest should be given as this will sustain them during the stressful time ahead.

The child may be disorientated or agitated as a result of the suddenness of the accident and because of the unfamiliar environment. This may be further compounded where the child is nursed in isolation and is another reason why the parents should be present whenever possible.

If the child is disorientated, the nurse should talk to him quietly and calmly, taking care to explain where he is and why. All procedures should be carefully explained in terms that the child can understand. The amount of detail and presentation of explanation will vary according to the child's age. If the child is agitated and frightened, the nurse must remain calm so that a relationship of trust develops between the child, his parents and the nursing staff.

The Post-shock Phase

Once hypovolaemic shock has been controlled, tangential excision of the injured area will be performed. This involves the surgical excision of necrotic tissue until viable tissue is encountered. The eschar is removed surgically to facilitate early application of skin grafts. These procedures reduce the risk of septicaemia and metabolic problems. The excision is usually performed in the operating theatre under a general anaesthetic within 72 hours of the injury.

Skin grafts must have small incisions in them to allow serum to be released, which is an aid to good graft taking. It is usual to nurse the child with the skin grafts exposed: this allows toileting of the wound two- to four-hourly during the first 24 hours. All serum must be expressed from beneath the grafts as this is one contributory factor to the failure of skin grafts to take. The donor site will be dressed with paraffin gauze, Videne or dry gauze and a pressure dressing, and must be observed for oozing of serum during the first 24 hours and repacked if necessary. The donor site should have healed within 10 days.

Infection   Infection is a major problem when extensive skin loss has occurred. The healing process is delayed because the infection creates further tissue destruction, which results in an increase of fibrous tissue formation. *Staphylococcus aureus*, *Pseudomonas aeruginosa* and the betahaemoleytic group A *Streptococcus* are the organisms commonly responsible for infection; if infection occurs, the appropriate systemic antibiotic is given. Meticulous attention to asepsis during the initial debridment procedure will aid in preventing infection. However, should infection become a problem, the nursing care will involve applying Videne to the affected areas on alternate days until wound swab culture is negative.

Nutrition   In severe thermal injury negative nitrogen balance causes increased metabolic requirements which may affect the child's chance of survival, and nutritional needs are met only with difficulty. The child may become unco-operative, anorexic and reluctant to eat the increased amounts of food required to correct the weight loss and reverse the catabolic state. Added to this is the problem that many children are used to convenience foods, and it is difficult to introduce a well-balanced diet when the child is feeling anxious and unwell. The following is intended as a guide that may be used to ensure that the child is adequately nourished during the post-shock period.

1.   The child receives nothing orally until bowel sounds are present (approximately 24 hours). A fluid regime is then begun gradually via a nasogastric tube.
2.   The fluid regime commences with clear fluids and progresses to 4 per cent dextrose and 0.18 per cent sodium chloride.
3.   If this is tolerated, half-strength milk is introduced, progressing to full-strength and then fortified milk. The amount to be given is calculated from the child's weight, as for maintenance fluids.
4.   An adequate intake of calories and protein is essential. For children who have sustained major injuries involving over 20 per cent loss of skin, this may be calculated as follows:
     Calories – 60 kcal/kg body weight + 35 kcal/percentage of body surface burnt/area of burn
5.   Supplementary milk feeds may be given via the nasogastric tube.

Other nursing actions that should be taken to ensure that the child is adequately nourished include:

1.   maintaining a record of the child's oral and calorific intake;
2.   discussing the child's food preferences with the family. It is important to note any racial or religious limitations;
3.   involving the dietitian in planning meals;
4.   ensuring that both child and parents understand the importance of an adequate diet;
5.   providing small, frequent meals. If the child's condition permits it, he should feed himself, but the nurse should set a time limit for self-feeding. When this has expired and the child has not finished, he requires assistance;
6.   allowing the parents to assist with feeding. This is one of the few needs with which mother can help. Parents can also bring food in.

Pain   Pain associated with thermal injuries is a major problem. The child quickly learns to associate fear with procedures giving rise to pain, for example wound care. More traditional methods of alleviating pain, such as the administration of morphine, are often unsatisfactory, and may induce nausea and vomiting, which causes an increased loss of body fluids and prevents the intake of food, thus affecting the nitrogen balance. The administration of Entonox has proved to be a safe and successful method of alleviating pain during wound care and encourages a positive outlook for recovery. With individualised care, the nurse should have established a good rapport with the child, which will facilitate giving the Entonox. Pain relief is also of benefit in that the parents will participate in the child's care more readily if he is not distressed during painful procedures.

Itching   As a result of destruction of sebaceous and sweat glands, and because of hyperaemia of the injured area, itching often becomes a chronic debilitating complication. The child may become irritable, especially during the night. As a result of this loss of sleep the child will be tired during the day, which may affect his rehabilitation, especially his educational and social activities.

If itching becomes a problem, the following nursing actions may be taken to give relief and to prevent skin breakdown from scratching:

1. The child should understand why itching occurs and the importance of not scratching.
2. The child's finger and toenails are cut short.
3. Lanolin cream may be applied to healed areas.
4. A cold wet compress may be applied to itchy areas.
5. If itching persists despite the above measures, an antihistamine drug may be prescribed.

Inhalation Injury This is a serious complication caused by the inhalation of fumes and smoke, which act as an irritant to the respiratory mucosa and lung tissue. This produces oedema with possible ulceration, which may give rise to airway obstruction that affects the gaseous exchanges in the lungs and may result in hypoxia and hypercapnia. The development of this injury may occur in three phases:

1. Respiratory distress with cyanosis, occurring soon after the injury.
2. Pulmonary oedema, occurring within 36 hours.
3. Pneumonia, developing in three to four days.

The child will require intubation, ventilation and a humid atmosphere until blood gases are within normal limits, and as pulmonary oedema is a predominant sign of inhalation injury, intravenous fluids must be carefully monitored. Chest physiotherapy is an integral part of the treatment to ensure that lung function is restored to normal as soon as possible. Frequent suction via the intubation tube is carried out to aid maintenance of the airway. Antibiotic therapy, when indicated, will be prescribed.

Psychological Trauma Psychological trauma following thermal injury is so damaging to the child and family that measures must be taken to alleviate the distress and aid acceptance of the disfigurement. The need to nurse the child in isolation further compounds this problem and is detrimental to the child's psychological and social development. The problem is particularly acute with children under 5 years of age because it is a time when a child should not be separated from his closest relative.

Fear is always a problem for the burnt child. It includes fright and anxiety about the accident and the agent that caused it, fear of sight of the injury and disfigurement, and guilt feelings.

To allay fear, all procedures should be explained and every opportunity given to the parents and their child to express their worries. The child's age will influence the effectiveness of verbal communication, and other methods of communication such as play may have to be used. The nursery nurse is a valuable member of the team, and through play she can help the child to express his fears and encourage him in all the care that will be necessary. The use of puppets has proved to be invaluable. The child identifies with these and, as a consequence, finds it easier to verbalise his fears.

Fright is sometimes manifested as disturbed sleep or nightmares. The following measures should help to ensure restful nights:

1. The child should be woken if he appears to be having a nightmare, and comforted, by talking to him and, if his injuries allow, cuddling him. A warm drink may be helpful.
2. The next day the child should be encouraged to talk about his nightmares.
3. If the problem persists, referral to a clinical psychologist may be necessary.

The child who has been grossly disfigured may be acutely distressed by his altered body image, and this may show as periods of loneliness or feelings of rejection from family or peers. Without support and counselling towards acceptance of an altered body image, such children may become self-imposed social outcasts who have difficulty in adapting to family life and may become school refusers.

The nurse who is faced with these problems should base care on the following actions:

1. She should introduce the subject of scarring gradually, allowing time for discussion and encouraging the child to touch his scars. She will be able to assess the extent to which the child is afraid of sibling, peer group and parental non-acceptance of his injuries. Where such fears exist, the nurse can overcome them by talking to the parents and siblings, showing photographs and allowing them to express fears of repulsion prior to visiting. Where the child's major fear is the acceptance of his gross disfigurement, continuous counselling, encouragement and support are necessary. From admission to hospital the child should be encouraged to discuss freely his injuries and any fears that he may have with the staff and his parents.
2. When siblings visit the child, the nurse and parents must be present to monitor reactions and discuss with parents any problems that may arise.
3. The nurse should visit the child's school prior to discharge from hospital to discuss his new appearance, showing photographs to teachers, classmates and friends. Again, fear of repulsion should be discussed to facilitate the injured child's return to school.
4. If the child has facial injuries and scarring, these problems may be amplified. The nurse should accompany the child to new destinations and stay with him until he feels secure. It is important that the child should be dressed in ordinary clothes (not pyjamas) wherever possible.
5. If adverse reactions from the public are experienced, the nurse and parents should discuss the reasons for this with the child. With patience and perserverance, this type of care should help the child to learn to live with his new body image and to cope with society's reaction to it.

The parents' main fear will be of touching the scar tissue, of the child's behaviour pattern and of how others, especially at school, will react to the child. In order that the parents can be supported through the psychological trauma, they must be involved in all aspects of their child's care. They should be helped to accept the ugly scars and learn to touch them without showing signs of repulsion, or else the child will interpret this as rejection. Multidisciplinary meetings between nurses, social workers, psychologists and parents are extremely valuable in helping to alleviate the parent's fears, particularly about the psychological trauma. The child will benefit from parental support and physical contact will help him to accept his scars when he sees that others can touch them and still love him.

The consequences of thermal injuries can be so severe that the guilt complex that parents may subsequently develop can be exacerbated. The parents will require constant counselling from admission onwards, perhaps for many years. This may take the form, initially, of individual counselling and proceed to group counselling with similar parents whose children are at different stages of care. A professional such as a nurse, psychologist or social worker may lead the group, which should be informal to encourage parents' free discussion of their problems. This type of group may eventually become a self-help group. Support must be continued for as long as the family needs help and encouragement.

Preparation for Discharge

As soon as the child is admitted, a rehabilitation programme should be planned. Again parental involvement is essential. The objectives of such a programme should be to:

1. assist the child and his family to accept the disfigurement;
2. reduce the psychological trauma and thus enhance the child's quality of life;
3. prepare the child for returning to family life.

The child must not be isolated for long periods and should be encouraged to socialise with other children in the unit as soon as possible. The physiotherapist will assist the child to gain mobility and regain his independence. The social worker should discuss any problems that the parents may have, such as financial difficulties and housing; this will assist the child's integration into the family and reduce parental stress.

Leaving hospital is a big step for both family and child, as there may be difficulty in re-adapting to family life. To help the parents to feel secure they should take their child home for the day once or twice before he is actually discharged. This will help him gradually to get used to a normal way of life and will prepare the parents for his return as they may fear that they cannot cope with caring for him alone. On returning to the ward the parents can discuss any problems that may have arisen and be given advice by the nurse and other members of the multidisciplinary team.

It is common after thermal injuries for the child to display behaviour problems such as school refusal. The nurse should advise the parents what types of behaviour to expect in their child after discharge and how to deal with them. The 12-year-old child shown in Figure 10.3 exhibited behavioural problems resulting from his altered body image after extensive scarring from a scald when he was two years old.

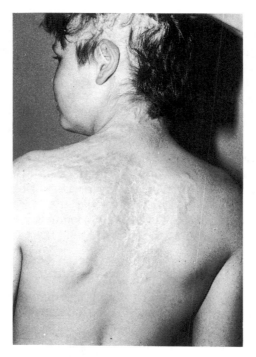

Figure 10.3 Widespread scarring after a
thermal injury, which resulted in behavioural
difficulties

After Care

An after-care burns clinic is an integral part of any burns and plastic surgery
unit. Such a clinic has a major role in providing continuity of care and support
for the child and his parents on an out-patient basis. Its use can also facilitate
early discharge home and prevent hospitalisation for children with minor
thermal injuries. After-care clinic staff are responsible for the management of
hypertrophic scarring as well as the long-term psychological effects of thermal
injury.

Hypertrophic Scarring

Another result of thermal injuries is the development of hypertrophic scars,
which appear when the dermis begins to epithelialise. Capillary budding forms a
rich vascular network, fibroblasts are laid down in the interstitial space and
collagen fibres form. The new collagen is not organised as before but is dense,
elastic fibres are not formed for many months and the scar is raised, red and
hard.

Hypertrophic scarring can be prevented by applying constant, uniform
pressure using a pressure garment. These garments help to reduce the formation
of scar tissue and thus the need for corrective and cosmetic surgery and the

hospitalisation that this would require. Good cosmetic results are produced, thus helping the child to accept his altered body image.

A pressure garment is manufactured to the individual child's measurements in flesh-coloured Lycra, which allows close approximation to the skin, so exerting constant, uniform pressure to the injured part. Areas such as the axillae and submental region require the use of extra pressure. The child will have to wear the garment for 23½ hours per day for at least 18 months, and if there are severe facial injuries, a hard facial mask underneath the Lycra pressure mask will also be required. As the child grows, new garments will be required. The garment should be removed three times daily while the child washes and to allow massaging of the injured area with Lanolin cream, which encourages the scars to become supple and reduces itching. Also, the child must have a daily bath. The garments must be replaced after treatment.

Small areas of breakdown may occur over the skin-grafted area and these may become infected, thus requiring a dressing; they will heal slowly as they are surrounded by new scar tissue.

The child should commence wearing a pressure garment within one to three months of the skin grafts healing. Both child and parents must be motivated towards correct wearing of the garment to achieve good results. The older child or adolescent often has difficulty in accepting the garment and will be self-conscious, particularly of facial masks. It is important, therefore, that both child and parents should understand how effective these garments can be in reducing scarring if worn correctly and continuously, and a positive approach by all concerned is essential to ensure that the child co-operates.

Prevention of Thermal Injury

As the thermally injured child and his family require care and support for many years after the initial injury, prevention of thermal accidents must have a high priority in the education of parents. Education and changes in the environment are both important.

Pre-school children are particularly liable to burns and scalds, and the health visitor is in an ideal position to educate and inform parents of the risk to their young children from thermal injuries. She should emphasise, on a one-to-one basis, the series of risks in the home, perhaps using a check-list such as:

1. Automatic fire (smoke) detectors should be installed in the house where feasible, and a fire blanket kept in the kitchen.
2. Cigarettes should be properly extinguished.
3. Thermostatically controlled deep fat fryers are advisable.
4. All fires must be adequately guarded.
5. Nightwear must be made from non-flammable material.
6. All bonfires and fireworks must be supervised by a responsible adult.
7. Household equipment should always be in good working order.
8. Cookers should have a wire mesh guard so that a child cannot pull a saucepan onto himself.

9. All saucepan handles should be turned inwards on cookers (but not to lie over heated rings).
10. The flexes of electric kettles and irons must not be within reach of young children. They should be kept short or coiled flexes should be used.
11. Cold water should always be run into the bath before hot.
12. There should be a reduction in the setting of hot water thermostats to a maximum of 54°C (which will give a 30-second safety margin before serious injury results).
13. Furniture made from non-flammable material should be used.
14. Matches should be kept out of the reach of young children.

It is important that parents should be able to administer first aid should a burn or scald occur in order to help to reduce the severity of the effects of the injury. First-aid information could be given through parentcraft classes or through publicity campaigns reinforced by health professionals. First aid information should contain the following points.

First Aid to Scalds

1. Immediately put the scald under cold water or run plenty of cold water over it to reduce the heat of the skin. It is important to do this for at least 10 minutes. Take off any clothes covering the scald so that the water can reach it.
2. Take off anything tight, such as a belt or jewellery, as scalded skin can swell.
3. Next, cover the scald with a clean, non-fluffy cloth, for example a clean cotton pillow case or linen tea towel. This reduces the danger of infection.
4. For anything other than a very small scald, the child should be taken to hospital, if necessary by ambulance.

Do not put butter, oil or ointment on the scald: it will have to be cleaned off again before treatment can begin. Do not prick blisters as this could lead to infection.

First Aid to Burns

Action to be taken against burns is the same as for scalds, except when burnt clothes are stuck to the skin: these should not be removed.

Publicity campaigns have had only limited success in preventing thermal injuries. One area in which there has been a worthwhile reduction in burns, however, has been with firework injuries, where there has been considerable media publicity for many years.

There have also been a number of successes for the environmental approach, sometimes combined with legislation. Before the introduction of flame-resistant nightwear for children by regulation, the plastic surgery wards were full of girls often horrifically burnt when their nightdresses caught fire. This problem is now quite rare. The use of guards on coal, gas and electric fires has also probably been one of the factors in the reduction of burns over the years, as has the more widespread use of central heating.

Many children still die in conflagrations caused by cigarettes igniting chairs and sofas. The regulations governing the flammability of upholstery are to be welcomed, but they have not been in force long enough to judge their effect.

References

Gaffin J (1981) Accidents in the home. *Nursing* (1st Series), **23**: 995–998.

Muir I F K and Barclay T L (1962) *Burns and their Treatment.* London: Lloyd Luke.

Recommended Reading

Artz C P Moncrief J A, Pruitt B A (1979) *Burns: A Team Approach.* London: W B Saunders.

CAPT (1987a) *Fact Sheet on Burns to Children.* London: CAPT.

CAPT (1987b) *Fact Sheet on Scalds to Children.* London: CAPT.

Fielden J *The Story of Kathy – a Burnt Child, by her Mother Jenny Fielden for Other Parents.* Opportunities for the Disabled, with the help of caring friends.

Jackson R H and Whittington C (1985) *Burn and Scald Accidents to Children,* Report of a Working Party of the Child Accident Prevention Trust. London: Bedford Square Press.

Martin H L (1970) Antecedents of burns and scalds in children. *British Journal of Medical Psychology,* **43**: 39–47.

Robinson S S (1968) Childhood burns in South Australia: a socio-economic and aetiological study. *Burns,* 5(4): 335–342.

Chapter 11
Poisoning
J R Sibert   Donna Mead

Four types of poisoning are seen in childhood: accidental ingestion of poisons in the under-fives, deliberate self-poisoning in older children, iatrogenic poisoning and non-accidental poisoning.

Accidental Child Poisoning

Accidental ingestion of poisons by younger children is a common problem. A typical story is that of a toddler who climbs up to get tablets while his mother's attention is directed elsewhere. Children accidentally ingest medicines, both prescribed and non-prescribed, household products and plants. The Home Accident Surveillance System estimates that, in 1986, 37 000 children aged from birth to four years and 3200 aged from five to 15 years attended Accident and Emergency Departments because of poisoning. Some children are also seen by general practitioners. A cohort study in New Zealand showed that 19 per cent of children had at least one incident of poisoning or suspected poisoning by the age of three years (Beautrais et al, 1981). No medical help was sought in many of these incidents.

Many children are sent home soon after their arrival in hospital because they have taken relatively non-toxic substances, and problems after accidental child poisoning are rare. Nevertheless, there are a few deaths every year from accidental poisoning: 74 children died between 1974 and 1983 in the UK. Other children, such as those with oesphageal stenosis following caustic ingestions, are left with serious problems after poisoning.

Aetiological Factors in Accidental Poisoning

The reasons why children should take a poisonous substance are intriguing, but there appear to be certain clues in the epidemiology of the problem. For instance, the sex ratio for poisoning in children is very similar to that for the general adult population, with boys and girls being approximately equal, in contrast to accidents as a whole, where the incidence in boys is much higher. Similarly, the social class of the families of poisoned children is similar to that of the general population, in contrast to other types of accidents where those to poorer families predominate. Indeed, there is some suggestion that the children of professional families may be more at risk of poisoning than others. The exploratory nature of a vulnerable age group, together with a lack of taste discrimination (especially around six to 18 months of age), may be a causative factor in some children.

Surprisingly, availability of poisons does not appear to be a major factor in accidental child poisoning. Baltimore and Mayer (1968), after a case control study, state 'there was no statistical significant difference between cases and controls on the number of storages of potentially toxic substances'. Sobel (1971) says 'contrary to common sense, frequency of poisoning is found to be unrelated to accessibility of poisoning substances'. Stress and behaviour problems within the family, however, do have a bearing on the problem.

One study in Cardiff (Sibert, 1975) showed that a number of stress factors were significantly more common in families with cases of poisoning than in controls (Table 11.1).

There is some evidence, too, that personality may play a part in the susceptibility of children to poisoning, with more hyperactive children being involved than might be expected by chance alone. It is difficult to be certain why stress is important in the aetiology of child poisoning; however, it is likely that child behaviour, even from such an early age, is altered in such circumstances. Parental attention may also be diverted at such times.

Table 11.1   Distribution of stress factors in poisoned and control groups

Stress factor	Families of children taking poison (n=100)	Control families (n=100)	χ^2	significant level
Serious family illness in last month	27	9	9.79	<0.002
Pregnancy	10	2	4.34	<0.004
Family house move within three months	12	1	8.23	<0.005
One parent away from home	18	5	7.07	<0.008
Anxiety or depression in parent	36	10	18.89	<0.002

Substances Taken in Accidental Poisoning

Children accidentally ingest medicines, both prescribed and non-prescribed, household products and plants.

Medicines   There has been a change in the pattern of poisoning admissions since 1976. In 1983, Lawson et al demonstrated that while the rate of admission for salicylate poisoning fell after the introduction of child-resistant containers (CRCs), the problem remained with other drugs, particularly benzodiazepines, tricyclic antidepressants and iron. These drugs are frequently prescribed for young mothers and, as such, are available in the houses of young children most likely to ingest tablets. Paracetamol remains a special case, for although CRCs were introduced for tablets in 1979, many children take paracetamol elixir, which has only recently been presented in CRCs. Luckily, however, serious paracetamol ingestion is uncommon in children, probably because the tablets are unpalatable and large, and the elixir sweet and sickly.

Table 11.2 shows the pattern of drugs ingested by children as described in the multicentre survey based at the Guy's Hospital Poison Unit (Wiseman et al, 1987).

Table 11.2   Drugs ingested by 1163 under-fives (data from Wiseman et al, 1987)

Class of Drug	Percentage of children
Analgesic	20
Other CNS drugs	14
Cough suppressant	12
Oral contraceptive	11
Anti-infective	9
Nutritional	8
Gastrointestinal	4
Bronchospasm relaxants	3
Ear, nose and throat preparation	3
Anti-allergic	3

Patterns of poisoning deaths in children in England and Wales have shown similar changes in admissions to hospital, with tricyclic antidepressants being the most common cause of death (26 cases between 1974 and 1980), followed by salicylates (eight), Lomotil (six), and quinine/chloroquine (five) (Craft, 1983). This is a change from the years immediately after the Second World War when salicylates were the most common substances involved in the deaths of children from poisoning.

Household Products   Household products are also commonly ingested by children. Many of the substances they take may be relatively non-toxic, but a few, such as caustic soda, soldering flux and paint remover, may cause serious harm. The numbers of children admitted to South Glamorgan and Newcastle hospitals over a nine-year period are shown in Table 11.3.

Substances that did not cause serious symptoms included bleach (89 cases), rat or mouse poison (53), disinfectant (43), perfume or aftershave (43), insecticide (33), cleaning fluids (28), nail varnish remover (22), window cleaner (21), shampoo (17), slug pellets (Metaldehyde) (13) and petrol (12).

Turpentine substitute and white spirit were the substances most commonly ingested. About 6 per cent of these children presented severe problems, with hydrocarbons tracking into the lungs and causing lipid pneumonitis. Paraffin is less commonly ingested in the UK, but is a very serious problem in the Third World, where children often drink it from jars thinking that it is water, not fuel.

Table 11.3 Poisoning from household products in South Glamorgan and Newcastle over a nine-year period (from Craft et al, 1984). Reproduced by kind permission of the *British Medical Journal*)

Household product	No. of cases	No. (%) with serious complications
Turpentine, white spirit or turpentine substitute	195	12 (6)
Paraffin	45	5 (11)
Alcohol	34	7 (21)
Paint remover	12	3 (25)
Sodium hydroxide (caustic soda)	10	8 (80)
Camphor oil	10	1 (10)
Resin hardener	3	1 (33)
Strong acids	2	1 (50)
Antifreeze	1	1 (100)
Soldering flux	2	2 (100)
Total	314	41 (13)

Alcohol is also a very serious poison for young children, with hypoglycaemia being a major problem, occasionally causing brain damage. Caustic soda ingestion may lead to serious oesophageal ulceration. Similarly, zinc chloride soldering flux leads to severe pyloric and gastric ulceration. Both may give strictures, as in the example of a two-year-old immigrant child who ingested soldering flux. She was initially well and was discharged home, but later presented with vomiting and failure to thrive. It was then found that she had a stricture of the pyloric region. She recovered well after operation.

Paraquat, the garden and commercial weedkiller, is a worrying poison because large doses cause pulmonary fibrosis, which is virtually untreatable. This problem is more commonly encountered when the commercial form rather than the much more dilute garden variety is ingested.

It must be remembered that most of the household products that children ingest do not cause serious symptoms. Bleach, in particular causes only minor symptoms, or oral erythema in a few instances, and serious cases are very rare.

A few children are admitted to hospital each year because they have ingested plants. Laburnum seeds are the most common plant poisons found in hospital admissions, and although some children have mild vomiting, serious problems are rare and death is virtually unknown.

In accidental child poisoning, as with other types of accident, three principal preventive strategies have been advocated. These are the use of educational campaigns, alterations in the environment and enforcement by law.

Educational campaigns aimed at removing unwanted medicines in circulation have often been advocated, but there is little or no evidence that these are effective. A campaign in Birmingham to publicise the problem and to encourage the return of medicines concluded that 'publicity, storage and destruction of unwanted medicines have little preventive value' (Harris et al, 1979). Ferguson et al (1982) in New Zealand evaluated placing 'Mr Yuk' stickers on poisons, together with a campaign, but this, again, had little effect on the incidence of admission after poisoning. The promotion of lockable medicine cabinets has been a feature of many education campaigns. Likewise, there is a dearth of evidence that these have been effective. It can be predicted that parents under stress would not remember safety education, that lockable medicine cabinets are possessed by a minority of households, and that parents under stress will not remember to use them.

One major success story in the prevention of childhood accidents is related to poisoning in children following the introduction of CRCs. It may be that part of the reason for the success of CRCs is because they do not rely on parental co-operation to be effective and should, therefore, be effective even in times of stress.

Regulations concerning the safer packaging of analgesics were introduced in 1976, and it has been shown by Jackson et al (1985) that hospital admissions for analgesic ingestion (of Junior Aspirin in particular) fell from 3884 in 1974 to 990 in 1978. The authors point out that there was a reduction in the ingestion of other poisons during the same period and suggest that this was due to a growing awareness of poisoning resulting from the debate over CRCs.

In 1978 CRCs were introduced by law for adult aspirin and paracetamol tablets. In 1982 a voluntary agreement was made between the Government and the Pharmaceutical Society whereby all prescribable solid-dose medications would be placed in CRCs or safety packaging, with exceptions for the elderly and infirm. Experience since 1982 has not been entirely encouraging (Sibert et al, 1985), and some pharmacists have not used CRCs. However, since January 1989 the Royal Pharmaceutical Society have made it a professional requirement for pharmacists to use CRCs in dispensing. In 1985 the Department of Trade and Industry agreed to put a number of household products, such as white spirit and turpentine substitute, into CRCs by regulation.

Regulations in the UK do not specify child-resistant closures alone: they also allow for blister and strip packaging. Until recently there has been little evidence on whether these blister packs are as effective as CRCs in preventing poisoning. Recently, however, a multicentre survey based at the Guy's Hospital Poison Unit (Wiseman et al, 1987) looked at the packaging of 938 medications taken by 877 children, compared to 5827 medications in control homes. Medications involved in suspected poisoning were most frequently packed in containers without child-resistant closures (63 per cent) or with transparent blisters (20 per cent). On the other hand, CRCs, strips, sachets and opaque blister packs all had low associations with poisoning incidents.

The pattern of accidental child poisoning has changed as a result of the withdrawal of Aspirin preparations for children, which occurred in 1986 because of the risk of Reye's syndrome, an acute inflammation of the liver and brain, which is often fatal. Paracetamol is now used instead of Aspirin.

Management of Accidental Poisoning in Childhood

Although the majority of children who present to hospital after accidental poisoning do not have serious symptoms, there are, nevertheless, a few children who have taken a significant poison and who are potentially or actually ill. It is clearly desirable to prevent unnecessary admissions to hospital, while maintaining safety. A way round this dilemma is to determine to which of four categories the substance the child has taken belongs: low toxicity, uncertain toxicity, intermediate toxicity or potential toxicity. After classification children can be either sent home, observed in the Accident and Emergency Department or admitted for observation or treatment. This approach is particularly relevant for the general practitioner as children who have taken substances of low toxicity (Figure 11.1) can be sent home and need not be referred to hospital.

Medicines	*Household products*
Antibiotics	Chalks and crayons
Antacids	Emulsion and water paints
Calamine	Fabric softeners
Oral contraceptives	Plant foods and fertilizers
Vitamins that do not contain iron	Silica gel
Zinc oxide creams	Toothpaste
	Wallpaper paste
	Washing powder (not Dishwashing powder)
Plants	
Begonia	
Cacti	
Cotoneaster	
Cyclamen	
Honeysuckle	
Mahonia	
Rowan	
Spider plant	
Sweet pea	

Figure 11.1 Substances of low toxicity when ingested

Older children who have taken poisons deliberately need to be treated differently. They should all be admitted to hospital for assessment, as should cases of iatrogenic and non-accidental poisoning.

The parents of all children who present with accidental poisoning should be given advice regarding storage of medicines and household products and the health visitor should, in all cases, be contacted to ensure this has been done effectively.

In many cases of poisoning in children, the stomach should be emptied in order to prevent absorption of the poison. This should usually be done by emesis using ipecacuanha paediatric mixture (Ipecac). This dose is 10 ml for six- to 18-month-old children and 15 ml for older children, and is followed by a tumblerful of water. The dose can be repeated after 20 minutes if necessary. There is evidence to suggest that Ipecac is more effective in removing toxic substances than is gastric lavage in children (Arnold et al, 1959; Boxer et al, 199). Ipecac is certainly more humane than lavage, which can be a distressing experience for a young child. The stomach should not be emptied in cases of hydrocarbon ingestion (such as kerosene or white spirit), or with caustic substances.

In the USA it has been argued that Ipecac should be kept in any home where there are young children, and many poisons centres in the USA recommend its use in this way. There have been cases, however, where Ipecac has been used inappropriately for caustic ingestion in the home. Despite this, it can safely be used in the general practice surgery for non-caustic, non-hydrocarbon poisons, particularly if there is a significant distance between the surgery and the Accident and Emergency Department.

Activated charcoal is being increasingly used in the management of poisoning in children because it absorbs toxic materials in the gut by offering alternative binding sites (Vale et al, 1986; Greensher et al, 1987). It is used either as an alternative to Ipecac or, more usually, after Ipecac-induced vomiting. Its routine use is limited by its poor acceptance by children, although it is particularly useful in tricyclic antidepressant poisoning.

If there is any doubt about the toxicity of a substance a child may have taken, a Poison Information Centre should be contacted day or night:

London – Guy's Hospital	Tel. 071-955 5095
Edinburgh – Royal Infirmary	Tel. 031-229 2477
Cardiff – Llandough Hospital	Tel. (0222) 709901
Belfast – Royal Victoria Infirmary	Tel. (0232) 240503

An important aspect of nursing care following accidental poisoning is to observe the child for progression of symptoms. When the central nervous system may be affected by the drug (e.g. with salicylate, barbiturate poisoning), the child should be observed for restlessness, confusion, delirium, convulsions and coma. When the respiratory system may be affected by the drug (e.g. benzodiazepines in very young children or diphenoxylate, the active constituent of the antidiarrhoea agent Lomotil), the child should be observed for signs of respiratory depression.

The nursing care of the poisoned child should involve not only the management of the poisoning itself, but also the recognition that accidental poisoning is an important symptom of family disturbance and stress. The nurse should make certain that an adequate psychosocial assessment is made, and if particular problems are highlighted, seek to involve other professionals. In all cases the health visitor should be involved.

It is considered that the health visitor's role is likely to be the most effective in achieving the objectives of preventing further episodes of poisoning. Research related to the efficacy of health education for prevention is far from definitive or conclusive. There is some evidence, however, to suggest that a correlation exists between perceived risks or recurrence and preventive health behaviour. This being so, the educational task of the health visitor is to enable the family to perceive the risks involved.

At the initial visit the health visitor will assess the family with particular reference to:

1.   family stress;

2.   family size (number of children) and support, if any, that the mother receives in child care, e.g. from the father or extended family;
3.   behaviour patterns of the children, with, for example, special reference to a hyperactive child or an adolescent;
4.   the availability and accessibility of medicines and other substances that may be accidentally or deliberately taken, in relation to points 1–3.

The information obtained at this assessment can then be used as a basis for predicting whether or not the risk of poisoning persists for any of the children in the family. If there is such a risk, the health visitor will arrange for follow-up visits and the necessary support.

One-to-one teaching for preventive health behaviour is known to be effective and, in this instance, would be warranted. Subsequent health education sessions might include:

1.   ensuring that the parents understand the importance of keeping medicines out of reach, or locked away when this is possible;
2.   ensuring that the parents are aware of the kinds of substances, e.g. white spirit kept in a pop bottle, or enteric-coated tablets that have the appearance of certain sweets, that may seem attractive to children;
3.   ensuring that the parents know what to do if accidental poisoning should recur, including the following:

   • act quickly
   • obtain help quickly
   • know how to obtain a GP or ambulance as necessary
   • know how to establish what and how much of a substance has been taken. If possible take the container and a sample of whatever has been taken to the clinic or hospital
   • do not give salt and water to make the child sick: salt can be harmful in large amounts;

4.   if a family member is taking medication regularly, e.g. a pregnant mother taking iron tablets, and if the health visitor feels that a child is at risk from poisoning, it may be possible to liaise with the GP who can ensure that the quantity of drug obtained with each prescription is limited. This precaution would be considered within the context of the distance between home and health centre and the parents' means of getting there.

The receiving of trigger factors or cues has also been shown to be effective in bringing about preventive health behaviour (Becker, 1974). Such cues may take the form of information-giving by health professionals. It can be seen, therefore, that by following a health education programme such as the one outlined subsequent episodes of poisoning may be avoided. (See also Chapter 2 for further information related to the health visitor's role in the prevention of childhood accidents.)

Deliberate 'Overdoses' in Older Children

Deliberate poisoning in older children forms one end of the age spectrum of 'overdoses' in adults. This occurs with emotionally disturbed children, usually following some psychological crisis. It is less common than accidental ingestion but needs to be taken seriously. A typical example is that of a girl in mid-puberty taking Valium tablets after a disagreement with her parents about going out with a boy. As with adults, a full psychiatric assessment is needed before discharge from hospital. Experience shows that such overdoses are often a symptom of a quite major problem at school, within the family or in the patient's reaction to his peers. Many substances may be taken deliberately by older children, and special attention has recently been focused on the increasing problem of drink in children of secondary school age. Like other types of deliberate poisoning, this may be a symptom of major psychological disturbance.

Glue Sniffing

Glue sniffing (solvent abuse) is another form of deliberate poisoning and has recently had a great deal of publicity. It is clear that in some adolescent subcultures, predominantly in working-class neighbourhoods, glue sniffing is the norm rather than the exception. Most solvent abusers are male adolescents who indulge in the habit as a group activity. Vale and Meredith (1981) reported that since 1970 there have been more than 50 deaths from solvent abuse in the UK. Admission to hospital because of solvent abuse is uncommon, but deaths are becoming more frequent and are usually associated with dangerous practices used during glue sniffing to increase euphoria – for instance solvent may be sprayed directly into the mouth, or a plastic bag with solvent inside it put over the head.

It is thought that neurological damage may occur after sniffing for less than a year and that symptoms may progress for up to three months after the habit has stopped. Clearly this is a form of deliberate poisoning that must be prevented.

The health professional's role in solvent abuse is a difficult one, which involves careful investigation of the underlying causes. An authoritarian approach should be avoided: the nurse's role in such abuse is to support and educate. Those most likely to be approached for help and advice are school nurses and health visitors, and the ward nurse if glue sniffing has lead to a hospital admission. The advice that should be given to parents who suspect that their child is abusing solvents will be considered in two categories:

1. Actual abuse.
2. Suspected abuse.

Actual Abuse   In an emergency and when the child is found unconscious, the solvent must be removed, the child's mouth and nose cleared, windows opened, an ambulance called and the hospital told what has happened. The parent or carer should try not to panic or become angry. Oxygen administration may be necessary.

If the child is still under the influence of solvent, he should be left until the effects have worn off, then asked calmly why he is involved in this activity, how often he does it and whether he does it alone or in company.

If the parents need help in understanding solvent abuse and appear initially reluctant to involve the social services department, they should be told of the existence of agencies such as 'Release' (Tel: 071-603 8654), which will act as mediator in such circumstances. It should be pointed out to parents that solvent abuse is not yet an offence for which the child will be taken to court, and also that they are not likely to be considered to be inadequate parents by those whom they approach for help.

Suspected Abuse   The increased incidence of children involved in glue sniffing is alarming, and most parents are aware of the possibility that their teenage children may engage in this activity. Their suspicions may be such that they will misinterpret the mood swings and irritability of adolescence for involvement in glue sniffing. It is important, therefore, that a parent who suspects that solvent abuse is occurring should be aware of the tell-tale signs:

1.   Glazed expression and slurred speech.
2.   The smell of the chemical on the breath.
3.   Inexplicable loss of appetite or weight.
4.   Lack of concentration on things that the child normally finds interesting.
5.   A sudden crop of spots around the mouth or nose.
6.   Small burns on the front of clothing where solvent has splashed.

It is important, however, to point out to parents that there could be many reasons for each of these signs. Confronting a child with an accusation that turns out to be ill-founded could prevent the parent from finding out what is really at the root of the child's abnormal behaviour.

'Release' provide a 24-hour information/referral service for parents and children who may want to talk about their problem. Confidentiality is ensured, but liaison with appropriate services can be arranged through the organisation's officials at the request of the client.

Prevention is by far the most important aspect of the management of solvent abuse, and every opportunity should be taken to educate teenagers about the serious short- and long-term hazards of glue sniffing.

Children sometimes take to glue sniffing out of boredom. Where this is the case parents should be advised to encourage their children to get involved in enjoyable activities, possibly with other members of the family, so that the risk of boredom is lessened. As a result of a recent Act of Parliament, traders are now not allowed to sell products containing solvents that may be inhaled to children under 16 years old. This is another example of enforcement being necessary to alter behaviour.

Non-Accidental Poisoning

Non-accidental poisoning has only recently become recognised as part of the spectrum of child abuse, in which the child usually presents with bizarre symptoms rather than poisoning. Why some parents choose to poison their children is difficult to know, but they often have a history of psychiatric disturbance and frequently have a paramedical background. Indeed, this problem forms one part of the 'Munchhausen syndrome by proxy', in which parents fabricate the signs and symptoms of disease in their child as a manifestation of their own psychological problems. Some examples may be helpful:

1.   An 18-month-old child presented with unexplained signs of unconsciousness – she had been given nitrazepam by her mother.
2.   A 10-month-old baby presented with pallor, vomiting and hyperventilation – she had deliberately been given Aspirin by her mother.
3.   A 2½-year-old girl presented with unexplained ataxia. She had had full investigation for a possible cerebral tumour before deliberate Phenytoin poisoning by her mother was discovered.

Such children should be dealt with under the child abuse procedure, as described in Chapter 14.

Treatment of Individual Poisons

If in doubt about the treatment or toxicity of a poison a child may have taken, Poison Centres throughout the UK are available for consultation and advice (see above).

Although the outcome of a poisoning is rarely fatal, great care needs to be exercised when there is any degree of uncertainty about the amount or type of product ingested.

It has been estimated that when children under five take medicines, the drugs concerned have, for the most part, been prescribed for mothers or grandparents. Poisoning normally occurs in the child's or grandparents' home following an episode (albeit brief) when the child has been left alone or accompanied only by another young child.

While education, particularly of parents and grandparents, undoubtedly has a significant role to play in the prevention of child poisonings, the major successful preventive measures are likely to be related to the environment and the production and packaging of the product.

Some common poisons taken by children, with notes on their toxicity and treatment, are given below.

Alcohol.   An increasingly commonly taken poison, especially by older children. It may cause severe hypoglycaemia, which should be detected by frequent blood glucose measurements, and prevented and treated by intravenous glucose infusions.

Antihistamines.   Do not usually cause significant problems in the quantities that children take.

Barbiturates.   Cause coma and hypertension. Forced alkaline diuresis may be needed in severe cases. This problem is getting less common, as barbiturates are less frequently prescribed.

Benzodiazepines.   Tranquillisers and hypnotics, such as diazepam (Valium), and nitrazepam (Mogadon), can cause drowsiness and coma, but problems are unusual. In very young children respiratory depression may need treatment with artificial ventilation, but this is rare in accidental ingestion.

Caustic Soda.   Can cause burns to the mouth and oesophageal ulceration, leading to stricture; review by oesophagoscopy and treatment with steroids has improved the outlook for this condition.

Digoxin.   Can be a serious poison in children, with only a few tablets being fatal. Cases should be monitored very closely, probably in an intensive cardiac unit, where ECGs are observed routinely. Beta-blockers, such as propranolol, should be used in severe cases, together with atropine where there is heart block. The serum potassium level should not be allowed to become too low or too high.

Diphenoxylate.   (The active constituent in Lomotil, the antidiarrhoeal agent.) This compound has an opiate-like action, which causes prolonged respiratory depression. Treatment is with the opiate antagonist Naloxone.

Iron.   Iron is a potentially very serious poison, initially causing vomiting and haematemesis, going on to acute gastric ulceration and shock. Later, however, convulsions and cardiac arrhythmias may occur. Iron tablets may be detected by X-ray of the abdomen.
    Treatment should be aimed at preventing further absorption of the iron by the use of chelating agents, such as desferrioxamine mesylate, instilled into the stomach, together with sodium bicarbonate solution. The same chelating agent should also be used parenterally (usually intravenously) in all cases where a potentially toxic amount of iron may have been taken.

Kerosene, Paraffin, White Spirit and Turpentine Substitutes.   Cause problems from aspiration into the lungs, leading to pneumonitis. Therefore vomiting should not be induced or lavage used. Treatment in mild cases is symptomatic, together with the use of prophylactic antibiotics. Corticosteroids are often used, but clear evidence of their effectiveness is lacking. Severe cases may need oxygen and intensive respiratory care.

Morphine and Related Opiates (Pethidine, Codeine, etc.).   Can cause respiratory depression. The use of the opiate antagonist Naloxone is recommended.

Paracetamol.   Serious poisoning is very rare in children. If it does occur, N-acetyl cysteine or methionine should be used.

Salicylates.   Severe poisoning is now rare. If it does occur, forced alkaline diuresis is used. Peritoneal dialysis may also be effective.

References

Arnold F J, Hodges J B, Barta R A, Spector S, Sunshine I and Wedgewood R J (1959) Evaluation of the efficacy of lavage and induced emesis in treatment of salicylate poisoning. *Pediatrics*, **23**: 286–301.

Baltimore C L and Meyer R J (1968) A study of storage, child behavioural traits, and mother's knowledge of toxicology in 52 poisoned families and 52 comparison families. *Pediatrics*, **42**: 312–317.

Becker M H, Drachman R H and Kirscht J P (1974) A new approach to explaining sick role behaviour in low income populations. *American Journal of Public Health*, **64**(3): 205–216.

Beautrais A L, Fergusson D M and Shannon F T (1981) Accidental poisoning in the first years of life. *Australian Paediatric Journal*, **17**: 104–109.

Boxer L, Anderson F P and Rowe D S (1969) Comparision of Ipecac induced emesis with gastric lavage in acute salicylate ingestion. *Journal of Paediatrics*, **74**: 800–803.

Craft A W (1983) Circumstances surrounding deaths from accidental poisoning 1974–1980. *Archives of Diseases in Childhood*, **58**: 544–546.

Craft A W, Lawson G R, Williams H and Sibert J R (1984) Accidental childhood poisoning with household products. *British Medical Journal*, **288**: 682.

Ferguson B A, Harwood C J, Beautrais M A and Shannon F T (1982) A controlled trial of a poison prevention method. *Pediatrics*, **69**: 515.

Greensher J, Mofenson H C and Caraccio T R (1987) Ascendency of the black bottle. *Pediatrics*, **80**: 949–951.

Harris D W, Karindiker D S, Spencer M G, Leach R H, Bower A C and Mander G A (1979) Returned medicines campaign in Birmingham, 1977. *Lancet*, **ii**: 599.

Jackson R H, Craft A W, Lawson G R and Sibert J R (1985) Changing pattern of poisoning in children. *British Medical Journal*, **287**: 1468.

Lawson G R, Craft A W and Jackson R H (1983) Changing pattern of poisoning in children 1974–81. *British Medical Journal*, **287**: 15–17.

Sibert J R (1975) Stress in families of children who have ingested poisons. *British Medical Journal*, **ii**, 87–89.

Sibert J R, Clarke A J and Mitchell M P (1985) Improvements in child resistant containers. *Archives of Diseases of Childhood*, **60**: 1155–1157.

Sobel R (1971) The psychiatric implications of accidental poisoning. *Pediatric Clinics of North America*, **17**: 653.

Vale J A and Meredith T J (1981) Solvent abuse. *Medical Education International*, **9**: 412–415.

Vale J A, Meredith T J and Proudfoot A T (1986) Syrup of Ipecac: is it really useful? *British Medical Journal*, **293**: 1321–1322.

Wiseman H M, Guest K., Murray V S G and Volans G N (1987) Accidental poisoning in childhood: a multicentre survey. *Human Toxicology*, **6**: 293–314.

Recommended Reading

Cameron J S (1988) *Solvent Abuse: A Guide for the Carer*: Beckenham: Croom Helm.

Oliver J S and Watson J M (1977) Abuse of solvents for kicks: a review of 50 cases. *Lancet*, **i**: 84–86.

Rogers D, Tripp J, Bentovim A, Robinson A, Berry D and Goulding R (1976) Non-accidental poisoning: an extended syndrome of child abuse. *British Medical Journal*, **1**: 793–796.

Scherz R G (1970) Prevention of childhood poisoning. *Pediatric Clinics of North America*, **17**: 713.

Sibert J R, Craft A W and Jackson R H (1977) Child resistant packaging and accidental child poisoning. *Lancet*, **ii**: 289–290.

Taylor E A and Stanfield S A (1984) Children who poison themselves. *British Journal of Psychiatry*, **145**: 127–135.

Chapter 12
Drowning
J R Sibert

Drowning is an important cause of accidental death in children, only deaths in road traffic accidents and from burns and scalds being more frequent. In 1987 47 children died from accidental drowning in England and Wales, as against 381 dying in road traffic accidents and 89 from burns (OPCS, 1988).

Many more boys than girls drown (40 to 13 in England and Wales in 1986), which presumably reflects the very different behaviour patterns of boys. There are also very heavy social class gradients, with disadvantaged children being more likely to drown. One mode of drowning that does not follow this pattern, however, is death in private swimming pools. This problem is particularly common in Australia where many families have their own pools.

The size of the problem of drowning and near-drowning in Britain has been virtually unknown, but it has been studied recently in Wales by Sibert et al (1987), observing children aged 14 years and under who either died from drowning or were admitted to hospital following a near-drowning episode. Information on near-drowning was obtained by personal enquiry of all consultant paediatricians in Wales. Between 1981 and 1984 36 children (25 boys and 11 girls) were admitted to hospital following near-drowning episodes. Five of these later died – four several days and one over a year after the incident. This boy and one other were left severely handicapped, confirming that children do occasionally survive near-drowning episodes but are left with severe brain damage.

Twenty-seven children (25 boys and two girls) died in the four years of the study, the majority drowning in rivers and lakes. In contrast, most of the children who nearly drowned were in swimming pools, and many had effective poolside resuscitation. The population of children aged 1–14 years in Wales in 1982 was 533 100; this gives an incidence of near-drowning in children in Wales of 1:60 000 children per year, and of drowning of 1:79 000 children. When boys alone are considered, the rates are 1:43 000 per year for both near-drowning and drowning. Drowning and near-drowning remains an under-researched field in the UK, with little work done on its causation, prevention and sequelae.

Emotional Sequelae

In families in which a child has died, whatever the cause, there is a high risk of marital breakdown. In keeping with this there is evidence of major emotional sequelae in the parents and siblings of drowned children. Nixon and Pearn

(1977), in keeping with many other studies of the effects on the family of a child dying, found that 24 per cent of parents separated following the drowning of their child; these authors comment, 'In one sense a child's death is more honourable, from society's point of view, if a child dies from a chronic medical illness, such as leukaemia. In the case of a child's death in the family bathtub or backyard swimming pool, the extra social sanctions of culpability and accusation further intensify the likelihood of the grief processes being transformed into a pathological variant.'

Causes of Drowning

Children can drown indoors or outdoors, in deep or shallow water. Some of the places where they can drown are shown in Figure 12.1. The possibility of non-accidental drowning must always be remembered, particularly in young children (Nixon and Pearn, 1977).

Indoors	*Outdoors*	
bath tubs	Natural:	sea and beaches
pails		rivers
baths and jacuzzi tubs		lakes, pools and ponds
indoor swimming pools	Manmade:	ornamental pools
		paddling pools
		public baths
		private swimming pools
		canals and drainage ditches

Figure 12.1 Some of the places in which children can drown

In Wales the majority of children who were admitted to hospital after nearly drowning did so after incidents in public swimming baths, and many of these children had had effective poolside resuscitation. In contrast, the majority of children who drowned did so in rivers, lakes and reservoirs, and were almost all older boys (Sibert et al, 1987). Unsupervised older boys in Australia were also found to be at risk of drowning in creeks (Nixon et al, 1986). A significant number of toddlers die in private pools.

Pathophysiology of Drowning and Near-Drowning

The excellent prognosis for some children rescued from apparent death (Pearn, 1977) has encouraged a better understanding of the pathophysiology of drowning. The majority of deaths from drowning, even among competent swimmers, occur within 10 m of a safe refuge. This suggests that some physiological disturbance, associated with the initial immersion, is in many cases responsible for incapacitation. There may, of course, also be some pathological reason why a child drowns. Orlowski et al (1982) have suggested that children with epilepsy may be four times more likely to drown than the general child population: this may be because children hyperventilate in cold water or before immersion, and this may induce a convulsion in a susceptible child.

The ability of diving mammals to remain under water, sometimes for up to 30 minutes, is due to a peculiar reflex, the 'diving reflex', in which the peripheral circulation is shut down with a profound bradycardia and the brain receiving the majority of the circulation. Man has a vestigial diving reflex, which is more marked in children and is exaggerated by cold and fear (Golden, 1980). It may be that the survival of some children after a long period of immersion is due to the diving reflex, particularly when there has been rapid cooling. Recently, however, it has been suggested that the diving reflex is not active in humans (Ramey et al, 1987). Harries (1986) has suggested that the reason some people survive prolonged periods underwater is because the circulation fails as a secondary event some time after immersion and because there is the protective effect of hypothermia. Orlowski (1988) has described this as 'ice water drowning', after a review of the literature revealed that all cases with a good outcome after very prolonged immersion occurred in water temperature of 10°C or less. This suggests also that it is the hypothermia that is protective.

Complications and Sequelae of Near-Drowning with implications for management

There is some controversy over how many children suffer severe brain damage (after being resuscitated) following a near-drowning episode. Evidence from Queensland, Australia, and Hawaii has suggested that the incidence of neurological deficit after near-drowning is 5 per cent or less. In Hawaii, for instance, in one study, 75 children were admitted to hospital having been apnoeic and unconscious after nearly drowning (Pearn et al, 1979). Of these, five died within seven days of rescue and the remaining 70 were neurologically normal on follow-up. In contrast, a study in California (Peterson, 1977) revealed that 21 per cent of children admitted after near-drowning were brain damaged. In the study in Wales (Sibert et al, 1987) severe brain damage occurred after near-drowning in the cases of two boys who were left with spastic quadriplegia, one after falling from a boat into the water and the other after falling into a swimming pool; both boys had had waterside resuscitation.

Clearly, it would be helpful to find out what factors are prognostic of severe brain damage in the nearly drowned child. Frates (1981) has analysed 42 cases of near-drowning in California and found that fixed and dilated pupils perfectly predicted those who would die or sustain permanent brain damage. He also noted that the prognosis was much worse when the near-drowning episode occurred in warm water. Preliminary results from an all UK study suggests that some children survive normally after presenting unconcious with fixed dilated pupils after near drowning (Kemp and Sibert 1990).

Many children who have had a severe hypoxic episode following near-drowning will develop cerebral oedema; this oedema may contribute to the ultimate brain damage suffered by these casualties.

Haemolytic Crisis There has been much discussion about the possible differences between salt and fresh-water drowning in children because of the potential, shown in experimental animals, for haemolytic crises following aspiration of large volumes of fresh water into the lungs. In practice much smaller volumes are aspirated by humans, and fears of haemolytic crisis have proved to be unfounded. It may be, however, that secondary drowning is more serious in salt water than in fresh water.

Aspiration Pneumonia A proportion of children who nearly drown aspirate water and develop pneumonia with secondary infection. This is rarely a serious complication unless the child has also developed brain damage.

Secondary Drowning Secondary drowning is a phenomenon in which respiratory deterioration occurs, with apparent pulmonary oedema, between one and 72 hours after the original incident. Harries (1986) suggests that this complication occurs only in the first 24 hours after the incident. Pearn (1980) has demonstrated that the problem occurs in children; he found that the victims in approximately 5 per cent of near-drownings were affected, and that there may be a worse prognosis in salt-water than in fresh-water near-drownings. The alveolar membrane dysfunction is probably due to surfactant deficiency, and is treated by adequate ventilation, usually by intermittent positive pressure ventilation (IPPV). The value of corticosteroids is unproven, but these are often given in treatment.

Treatment of Drowning

The aims of treatment of an immersion victim are to restore adequate ventilation and circulation, prevent further heat loss and correct acid/base status. Apart from directly correcting the acidosis, these can usually all be achieved at the waterside. Simple first aid with mouth-to-mouth resuscitation, covering and warming are vital. Many children vomit during resuscitation, so it is important to ensure a clear airway throughout the resuscitation procedure. The question of which children should be resuscitated at the waterside is made difficult because of the conflicting evidence from the literature on brain damage and near-drowning. However, in view of the fact that some apparently dead children may recover fully from near-drowning episodes (Pearn, 1977), it is wise to attempt to resuscitate all apparently dead, drowned children. This is particularly so in cold water drowning.

All children who may have inhaled water should be admitted to hospital. The presence of lung crackles audible on direct auscultation of the chest is helpful in deciding whether or not there has been aspiration. Those children who have adequate ventilation and no apparent sequelae should be reviewed for 24 hours for signs of secondary drowning and supraventricular cardiac arrhythmias. They should also be given chest physiotherapy. Secondary drowning should be treated by positive end expiratory pressure (PEEP) ventilation.

Severely ill children who cannot initially maintain adequate oxygenation should be admitted to the intensive care unit where they can be mechanically ventilated. The management of such children has been reviewed by Golden (1980). Those children who show neither respiration nor cardiac output should be ventilated, have external cardiac massage and have their acidosis corrected. Respiratory acidosis is corrected by mechanical ventilation, whereas metabolic acidosis is corrected by administration of sodium bicarbonate. If the core temperature is below 28°C, consideration should be given to slow rewarming. The effect of hypothermia, previously standard barbiturate therapy and regulating the intracranial pressure, with monitoring, on hypoxic/ischaemic brain injury has been studied by Bohn et al in Toronto (1986). They found that these measures provided little benefit and recommended that therapy should be directed towards maintaining cerebral perfusion and adequate oxygenation.

Prevention of Drowning

Education

With prevention of drowning, there is probably more evidence of education and training being effective than with any other type of childhood accident. To be unable to swim increases the risk of drowning in childhood, and clearly it is advantageous if as many people as possible can swim. Indeed, there is evidence that teaching children to swim may have reduced the number of deaths among 5–14 year olds (Graham and Keating, 1978). Certainly, there has been an overall fall in the number of deaths in children from drowning that has coincided with better swimming training. Studies in Australia and the UK have shown that a number of older children drown while swimming unsupervised in rivers, lakes and creeks: this unsupervised swimming should be discouraged.

A number of children die each year in public swimming pools; at least some of these deaths could be prevented by better supervision at the poolside. This should remain a high priority for local authorities, and health professionals should be able to lobby them on this issue. Children can also drown in ornamental pools, and families with young children are well advised to fence or cover these. The health visitor is in an ideal position to comment on this aspect of home safety during a visit. Life jackets and buoyancy aids are important in helping to prevent children in boats and canoes drowning should they fall overboard. Getting children to wear them is a difficult problem, and education of parents is important. Boat and canoe clubs can insist that their members wear them.

Environmental Measures

There are a number of environmental measures that can help to prevent drowning. Private swimming pools are a significant hazard in warm, affluent countries such as the USA and Australia; they cause about seven deaths per year in the UK, mostly of toddlers (Barry et al, 1982). There is good evidence that fencing that prevents children from having access to pools can prevent drowning. Pearn and Nixon (1977) compared drownings in private swimming pools in Brisbane and Canberra. In Canberra swimming pools have, by law, to be fenced, but there is no such legal sanction in Brisbane; only one child died in the Australian capital from a swimming pool accident over a five-year period, compared with 55 in Brisbane. We still await any such legislation in the UK.

References

Barry W, Little T M and Sibert J R (1982) Childhood drownings in private swimming pools; an avoidable cause of death. *British Medical Journal*, **285**: 542–543.

Bohn D J, Biggar W D, Smith C R, Conn A W and Barker G A (1986) Influence of hypothermia, barbiturate therapy and intracranial monitoring on morbidity and mortality after near-drowning. *Critical Care Medicine*, **14**: 529–534.

Frates R C (1981) Analysis of predictive factors in the assessment of warm-water near-drowning in children. *American Journal of Diseases in Childhood*, **135**: 1006–1010.

Golden F (1980). Problems of immersion. *British Journal of Hospital Medicine*, 373–376.

Graham J M and Keating W R (1978) Deaths in cold water. *British Medical Journal*, **2**: 18–19.

Harries M (1986) Drowning and near-drowning. *British Medical Journal*, **293**: 123–124.

Kemp A and Sibert J R Annual Meeting of British Paediatric Association 1990.

Nixon J and Pearn J H (1977) Emotional sequelae of parents and sibs, following drowning or near-drowning of a child. *Journal of Psychiatry*, **11**: 265–268.

Nixon J, Pearn J, Wilkey I and Corcoran A (1986) A fifteen year study of child drowning. *Accident Analysis and Prevention*, **18**: 199–203.

Office of Population Censuses and Surveys (1988) Deaths from accidents and violence. *Quarterly Monitors* DH4 Series 1988.

Orlowski J P, Rothner A D and Lueders H (1982) Submersion accidents in children with epilepsy. *American Journal of Diseases in Childhood*, **136**: 777–780.

Orlowski J P (1988) Drowning, near-drowning and ice water drowning. *Journal of the American Medical Association*, **260**: 390–391.

Pearn J H (1977) Neurological and psychometric studies in children surviving fresh-water immersion accidents. *Lancet*, **1**: 7–9.

Pearn J H (1980) Secondary drowning in children. *British Medical Journal*, **281**: 1103–1105.

Pearn J H and Nixon J (1977) Are swimming pools becoming more dangerous? *Medical Journal of Australia*, **1**(8001): 7–9.

Pearn J H, Bart R D and Yamaoka R (1979) Neurological sequelae after childhood near-drowning. A total population study from Hawaii. *Pediatrics*, **64**: 187.

Peterson B (1977) Morbidity of childhood near-drowning. *Pediatrics*, **59**: 364.

Ramey, C A, Ramey D N and Hayward J S (1987) Dive response of children in relation to cold water drowning. *Journal of Applied Physiology*, **63**: 665–668.

Sibert J R, Webb E & Cooper S (1987) Drowning and near-drowning in children in Wales. *Practitioner*, **232**: 439–440.

Chapter 13
School Injuries
Julia Walsh

A significant proportion of childhood injuries occur in school, which Hodgson et al (1984) describe as the primary workplace of the young. Unfortunately school injuries, which are a serious health issue, have not always received the appropriate attention. It must be recognised that accidents at school are an important health hazard and improvement is needed in all areas of education and injury management of the staff concerned. School nurses can play an integral role in seeing that this improvement is made.

The role of the school nurse, and her job description, varies considerably from health authority to health authority and to a certain extent also depends on how she as an individual may develop her job. She may be based in one school and serve that school and several others, be based at a clinic and serve several schools, or be based at and serve one school only. The ages of the pupils she may have to deal with can range from 5–18 years. Her qualifications may vary from EN to RGN with RSCN or HV(Cert), and she may also have undertaken an optional specialised school nurse course.

There are nationwide variations in local education policies toward health and safety. Some education authorities employ school matrons whose primary task is to care for injured or unwell children at individual schools. Other authorities expect school helpers, secretarial and teaching staff to care for these children. Children with special needs, for example the physically disabled, usually have a care assistant assigned by the education authority to care for them individually, either in a 'normal' school or as part of a group in a 'special' school.

The Role of the School Nurse

The school nurse may have three roles in relation to accidents that occur at school – to prevent such accidents, to educate, and to liaise – none of which is dominant and all of which are important in their own way and overlap with one another. The nurse can also be seen as having several client groups: school staff, pupils and parents.

The School Staff

The responsibility for dealing with accidents is such that the school nurse may be involved in giving advice on the situation and quality of first aid and treatment only. Of particular importance, however, is prevention and the training of staff. The nurse's advice may be sought on aspects of a programme of accident prevention and safety education, and she may be involved in taking an active part in such a programme (see 'An Integrated Plan of Health Education in Accident Prevention' below).

An important part of her work as a liaisor is as a source of information on the health of the school's pupils, because ill health may, in certain circumstances, put some children at risk of accident; for example, a child with epilepsy should not go swimming unless closely supervised. The school nurse should maintain her accident prevention role by recording the injuries that occur at school and, in conjunction with the school staff, identifying areas and activities of particular risk, for example sniffing glue and other noxious substances. She may also be involved in giving staff first-aid instruction and promoting awareness of safety, being aware of and reinforcing the school's safety rules. A two-way exchange on all these issues should be encouraged between staff and pupils.

Although the immediate task of the school nurse is to prevent accidents, her responsibilities as an educator involve turning out safety conscious individuals better adapted to the hazards of modern life.

The Parents

The parents of a child who may be open to an increased risk of injury at school do not always recognise the need to tell the staff about it. The school nurse, in her privileged position as the recipient of such information, may outline the advantages of communication and thereby help to promote a liaison between staff and parents. She may consider it important to give support to parents of recently injured children when they return to school, advising on any special provisions that may have to be made to accommodate them. It may be advantageous to put parents in touch with those whose children suffer similar conditions, or give them information about agencies where monetary help may be sought.

The liaison between school nurse and staff may be used as a method of conveying information about parents' real or imagined fears regarding injuries at school, and the nurse may then be seen to be a link between home and school on health matters, which again will encourage better communication between staff and parents.

Liaison with Other Professions

In a preventive role, the school nurse may be involved at the planning stage of a new school or a new medical facility in a school. She should, therefore, have some knowledge of the facilities that should be made available to care for an injured child and of the safety factors that should be incorporated into the design of any new building. The school nurse usually hears about an injury to a child directly from the school or through a hospital discharge advice note. Liaison with hospital staff concerning a seriously injured child is beneficial, and a written report from ward staff may be particularly useful.

In a particular case of injury it may be decided to call upon the school medical officer to examine the child and recommend appropriate treatment and care; such decisions are usually taken after discussion between all concerned – school staff, parents, school nurse and sometimes the child himself. Other health professionals, such as the health visitor, GP, paediatrician, physiotherapist, ophthalmologist, speech therapist, chiropodist and audiometrician, may also be called upon. On the educational side, the home tutor service may be required until the child is able to return to school, which should be as soon as possible as the child will miss the social contact of school life.

In all these liaisons and exchanges of information, care should be given to the need for confidentiality: information given in confidence should not be passed on without the knowledge of the parents and the child.

Causes and Recording of School Injuries

There is very little statistical information on the cause of accidents in schools. There are no official methods of collecting overall information, although accident books have to be kept by staff. Accurate data on the size and nature of the problem would lead to the identification of hazards and, it is to be hoped, to the prevention of accidents.

The most recent official survey was undertaken by the Department of Education and Science (DES) in 1965. The survey investigated all school accidents leading to at least a half-day's absence from school that occurred within 10 local authority areas in England and Wales over three school terms. In this survey the playground, as might have been expected, was found to be the most common site of accident occurrence, with playing fields and the gym coming next in frequency. Relatively few accidents occurred in the classroom.

Very similar findings to these have been reported in a study in South Glamorgan in 1977 (Maddocks et al, 1978) by the South Warwickshire Health Authority (Avery and Parkin, 1982) and in a recent study funded by the Child Accident Prevention Trust in the Brighton Area. In this latter survey of just under 10 000 children presenting to Accident and Emergency Departments, 18 per cent of the injuries were incurred in school (in 22 per cent of school-age children). Of these children, 45 per cent were injured in the playground, while only 14 per cent of the children's time was spent there. Many of the accidents were the direct result of poor behaviour, and the authors speculated that increased teacher supervision at playtime might be beneficial in some schools.

No child can be completely free from risk in the school environment. Safety does not mean the elimination of all risk: some risks are inevitable, even necessary, but needless risks can be eliminated. Safety in the school does not imply that the physical environment be converted into an accident-proof cocoon or that children's actions be completely restrained so that accidents cannot happen. Rather, it means pursuit of the normal demands of life in an environment in which hazards are reduced to a practical minimum and the behaviour of pupils is adapted to safe and effective living. However, there is now concern about certain school leisure and games activities. Children have died on mountain and hill-walking expeditions in bad weather, and very close control needs to be kept on these activities by head teachers. Similarly, certain sports, particularly rugby football, may involve risk of neck and other injuries if teams of unequal size play together.

The data relating to fatal and major injuries in educational establishments have, since 1 January 1981, been directly reportable to the Health and Safety Executive (HSE) under the Notification of Accidents and Dangerous Occurrences Regulations 1980. Seventeen fatalities, 15 involving children, have been reported since then, illustrating a wide range of hazards that may arise.

Some well-identified hazards are uneven playground surfaces, unprotected or ill-maintained playground and sports equipment, electrical and other specialised equipment, sharp instruments, heavy furniture and classroom chemicals. School buildings have in recent years been planned to remove the cause of some accidents, especially those involving unsuitable flooring, glazing, dangerous obstructions and projections, and poorly planned circulation. Well-designed furniture, glare-free lighting, comfortable temperatures and a reduction in noise levels also help in the creation of a safe environment (DES, 1979). Unfortunately, many schools have inherited their buildings from another, less well planned and more hazardous era.

The Health and Safety at Work Act 1974

There are four parts to this Act, Parts 3 and 4, in the view of the HSE, being applicable to pupils in schools. Part 3 is concerned with the law relating to building regulations and Part 4 contains a number of miscellaneous and general provisions. One of the objectives of the Act is to safeguard people other than employees who may be affected by activities at places of work. The general standard of protection by an employer of an employee should be the same as for visitors and others within the workplace.

It is the duty of the *employer* under the Act:

- to ensure that machinery and systems are safe;
- to provide training, information and supervision for employees to ensure health and safety at work;
- to keep the place of work in a safe condition;
- to ensure health and safety of the environment and to protect safety policies.

In the realms of education the employer is the local education authority, which also acts as the enforcing body. It can be argued that different criteria should be applied to the general standards of protection in the field of education in view of the fact that the very young or the disabled may be more vulnerable than others and that they may be less knowledgeable about potential hazards.

It is the duty of the *employee* under the Act:

- to take every care over the health and safety of himself and of people who may be affected by what he does or fails to do at work;
- to co-operate with his employer where duties or requirements are imposed on the employer.

The Act also requires that all people at work and members of the public, including children, should not intentionally interfere with or misuse anything that has been provided to safeguard their health, safety and welfare.

In 1975/76 the HSE conducted a pilot study that demonstrated the impact of the Act upon educational activities and concluded that the local education authority held most of the legal responsibilities under the Act (HSE, 1975/6).

Following inspection of various educational establishments by the HSE Inspectorate, many schools were found to be relatively safe and had made active efforts to increase safety awareness. However, some local authorities had not produced an adequate safety policy (HSE Annual Report, 1982). The Education Service Advisory Committee set up in 1981 is a useful forum for the assessment of risk and, most importantly in times of financial constraint, for identifying priorities (HSE Annual Report, 1979). This committee has also set up working groups on safety policies and accident statistics, on training in health and safety and on the distribution of information and guidance. It has been suggested that the greatest contribution to health and safety in educational establishments will come from better training, greater safety awareness and improved methods of work, rather than from the provision of safety hardware (HSE Annual Report, 1980).

Two other sets of regulations that also have a bearing in the educational field are the Safety Representatives and the Safety Committee Regulations 1977 and the First Aid at Work Regulations 1981.

Prevention of Accidents in Schools

Not all accidents can be anticipated and it would be very difficult to foresee all situations that cause them. However, most hazardous conditions can be recognised and unsafe practices detected if a school has a well-organised safety programme. The following check-list (Creswell et al, 1976; reproduced by kind permission of Times Mirror/Mosby College Publishing) is one that could be adapted for use in most schools.

Reporting of Accidents
1.   Are accident report cards or forms available?
2.   Is there a complete written report on file for every accident that results in an injury?
3.   Is a special study made of the causes of each accident?
4.   Is an adequate follow-up made after each accident analysis to prevent recurrence of the accident?
5.   Is a rapid inspection made of the building each morning and a thorough inspection each month?

Gymnasium, Pool and Locker Rooms
1.   Is equipment in good condition?
2.   Are all exposed projections covered?
3.   Is the floor treated to prevent it from being too slippery?
4.   Are doors of a safe type?
5.   Are rules for the use of the gymnasium posted and practised?

6. Are pupils properly dressed for gymnastic activities?
7. Is horseplay prohibited?
8. Is unsupervised use of the gymnasium and pool prohibited?

Corridors and Stairs
1. Are all obstructions removed?
2. Are the floors and stairs treated to prevent them from being slippery?
3. Are worn or broken stairs replaced?
4. Are railings provided so that every person using the stairs can hold a railing?
5. Is undue congestion of corridor traffic prevented?
6. Are horseplay and running in corridors prohibited?
7. Are stairs taken one step at a time?

Laboratories and Home Economics Rooms
1. Is all equipment in good repair and inspected frequently?
2. Are all possible safety devices and attachments available and used?
3. Are lighting and space adequate?
4. Are safety rules posted and practised?
5. Are pupils properly instructed in the use of equipment?
6. Are horseplay and running prohibited?
7. Is the unsupervised use of laboratories or home economics rooms prohibited?
8. Are first-aid supplies immediately available?

Classrooms and Lecture Theatres
1. Are all obstructions removed?
2. Are exposed projections covered?
3. Are sharp objects placed in protected places?
4. Are radiators and electric fixtures properly protected?
5. Are dropped objects picked up immediately?
6. Is an orderly routine followed, with rushing and pushing prohibited?

Playground
1. Is apparatus in a safe condition and checked regularly?
2. Are children taught the proper use of each piece of apparatus?
3. Is supervision always provided when the playground is used?
4. Do the children assume co-operative responsibility for playground safety?

Athletics
1. Is approved equipment used?
2. Is competent supervision always provided?
3. Are the participants properly trained and sufficiently skilled?

Fire Protection
1. Are vacant rooms, basements and attics free from flammable material?
2. Is there proper insulation between heating equipment and inflammable material?

3. Are there two or more exits from every floor, with doors swinging outwards?
4. Are there adequate fire escapes on buildings of two or more storeys?
5. Are fire extinguishers of an approved type provided in sufficient number?
6. Are fire alarms centrally located?
7. Are fire drills so proficient that the building can be emptied in an orderly manner in less than three minutes?

Going to and from School
1. Are road crossings properly patrolled?
2. Are intensive studies made of the hazards that children may encounter going to and from school, and is appropriate action taken?
3. Are specific routes outlined for the pupils?
4. Are those who travel by bus given instruction on entering and leaving the bus as well as on conduct in the bus?
5. Are bicycle riders given proper instruction?
6. Are the parents enlisted in the safety programme to and from home?

An Integrated Plan of Health Education in Accident Prevention

Education in safety has two aims: to teach children to distinguish between which risks to take and which to shun, and to instruct them how best to deal with inevitable risks (Guillen, 1967). A successful education programme, therefore, would involve ensuring that all concerned be made aware of their specific roles and responsibilities toward accident prevention.

The Staff Individual schools should be the main instigators of accident prevention and safety awareness. The school nurse, the British Red Cross Society or the St John Ambulance Association, the road safety division of the police force and the local fire brigade may then be called upon to add their expertise in specialised areas. Representatives from each of these groups should be encouraged to meet and plan how their different areas of teaching can complement one another.

Informal talks with the staff, allowing time for discussion and questions, can be most productive. Here, topics such as accident-proneness may be discussed, so that health aspects may be understood by all the staff. With the increased integration of handicapped children into 'normal' schools, there will be a greater need for staff awareness of the increased risk of accidents to these children and of the special protective measures that may have to be employed, e.g. the wearing of protective headwear by a severely epileptic child.

Individual cases may be discussed with the relevant members of staff. In practice, however, it may be possible to inform only the head teacher or the department head and rely on them to pass the information on.

School staff should use local school rules to implement some safety measures; for example, methods of trafficking, creation of 'out of bounds' areas and restrictions on type of hairstyle, footwear and clothing may be used in an effort to prevent collisions, falls, slipping, tripping and occlusion of vision. In developing such rules it is important to bear in mind that the school is *in loco parentis* while the child is in school (Ireland, 1979). It is also important to remember that compliance with rules is more likely if pupils and parents understand the need for them.

Safety precautions necessary in practical teaching areas are probably best dealt with at the time of the lesson by the teacher concerned. Excellent publications (e.g. ROSPA, 1980) exist to assist teachers in dealing with the specific safety precautions for outdoor pursuits, in science laboratories and in practical and physical education. As previously stated, many injuries are the result of falls and collisions in the playground. Games developed to promote the ability to avoid, or minimise the result of, such accidents may be particularly useful and can be played in the physical education session (Figure 13.1). The need for vigilant supervision is paramount.

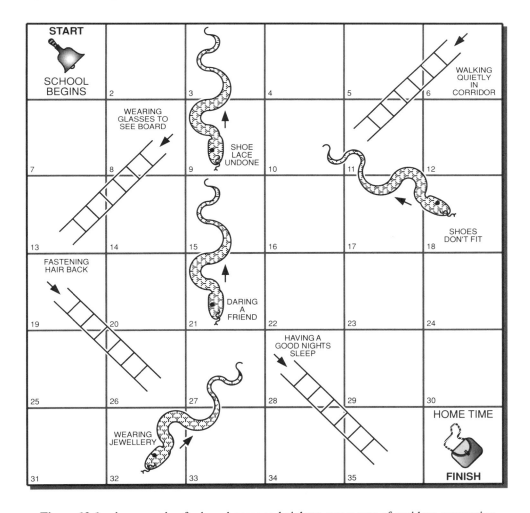

Figure 13.1 An example of a board game to heighten awareness of accident prevention

The Pupils   Accident prevention may be discussed in general terms as part of a group, or in more specific terms in a one-to-one relationship. The school child may view the topic very differently if the school nurse is involved, perhaps less as a teaching situation and more as a pattern of life, especially if she uses techniques designed to change attitudes. For a successful result, she should be well known and well regarded at the school.

A small group of younger children may benefit from a short introductory talk about accidents, followed by a discussion period so that they may share their experiences with the group. The causes of accidents may then be more graphically illustrated by the playing of games. Snakes and ladders, observation, card and true-or-false games may all be devised with safety as their themes (see Figure 13.1). Competitions may be devised for children to illustrate a particular safety theme or to create a slogan for an illustration or poster. Guillen (1967) advocates the use of a safety squad to involve the children in the general observation of their environment and to make them aware of any hazards that may be in it.

It will be seen that some of these methods may be too lengthy to include in one session with the school nurse but, by liaison with the teacher, it may be possible to carry them over into the normal school day: a new safety theme may be illustrated each week. In these safety sessions the causes of some specific accidents that may result in injury can be pointed out, for example: the unsafe wearing of clothing; untied shoe laces; badly fitting shoes; scarves and coats worn around the neck and used in games; a poor regard for the body's welfare (e.g. becoming physically unfit or not wearing aids or protective clothing when required); poor attitudes towards safety; failure to realise how they may put themselves and others at risk of an injury by their actions; and poor attitudes towards the environment (failure to realise their contribution towards an unsafe environment, e.g. the unsafe disposal of glass). The older child may be able to understand further specific causes such as the role of aggression in the causation of accidents.

On a one-to-one basis, accident prevention may be discussed quite spontaneously. It may not necessarily be undertaken at school and can easily be dealt with at home and also thereby gain the approval and co-operation of the parents. An informal approach, with time for questions and answers, is probably best.

Specific advice may need to be given here to a child who has a record of frequent injuries or 'near misses', and it may be necessary to try to discover the reason for this. A child with a well-identified additional risk of injury could be counselled using this method.

The Treatment of School Injuries

The role of the peripatetic school nurse in the treatment of injuries is largely advisory because she is rarely in the position of being able to render first aid. In general, when a school welfare assistant or the matron is responsible for dealing with accidents, reasonable facilities and treatment are available. These may include a separate first aid/medical room, a good, well-stocked first-aid box, a trained person always in attendance and comprehensively kept records of injuries. Liaison with the health and safety representative in schools may sometimes be rather poor where secretaries or school helpers have to treat accidents, and the provision of facilities is often less satisfactory, with no separate first-aid room, indifferent first-aid provision and, at times, completely untrained people dealing with accident care.

The majority of accidents in schools are minor, and in the main need a sympathetic attitude and the common sense that would be employed by most responsible adults. School staff are not encouraged to deal with anything but elementary first aid and are instructed to refer anything other than this through the parents to the local Accident and Emergency Department or health centre.

However, in some situations immediate and drastic initial treatment is vital and should be dealt with by a well-trained person, with a well-stocked first-aid box immediately to hand. Although a trained first aider is on the staff of many schools, he may not be available in every case. The training that he should have undergone may not have been recent, and argument suggests the need for retraining every three years.

The case for a separate first-aid room is perhaps more difficult to make, but the absence of the most basic facilities of hot water, paper towels and a chair or couch on which the child can recover in relative quiet should, however, justify its provision. Liaison between school staff treating injuries and the safety representative at the school should be close, so that the regulations concerning safety at school may be explored and staff and first-aid provision will be of an acceptable level.

It must be recognised that school injuries are an important health hazard and improvement must be made in areas of education and injury management. School nurses can play an integrated role in seeing that these improvements are made.

References

Avery J G and Parkin D (1982) *Childhood Accidents in South Warwickshire – a One Year Study in a Mixed Urban and Rural Environment*. Warwickshire: South Warwickshire Health Authority.

Creswell W H Jr, Newman I M and Anderson C L (1985) *School Health Practice*, 8th edn. St Louis: Times Mirror/C V Mosby.

Department of Education and Science (1979) *Safety at School: General Advice*, 2nd edn., Safety Series No. 6. London: HMSO.

Guillen E (1967). *Safety Games and Exercises*. London: G Bells & Sons Ltd.

Health and Safety Executive (1975/6) *Health and Safety in Schools and Further Education Establishments*. Pilot Study. London: HMSO.

Health and Safety Executive. Annual Reports 1979, 1980, 1982. *Manufacturing and Services Industries*. London: HMSO.

Hodgson B W, Woodward C A and Feldman W (1984) A descriptive study of school injuries in a Canadian region. *Paediatric Nursing*, May/June: 215–219.

Ireland K (1979) *Teachers' Guide to the Health and Safety at Work Act*. Kettering: School Masters Publishing Co.

Maddocks G B, Sibert J R and Brown B M (1978) A four week study of accidents to children in South Glamorgan. *Public Health*, **92**(4): 171–176.

Royal Society for the Prevention of Accidents (1980) *The Facts about Accidents* (SE62). Birmingham: ROSPA.

Recommended Reading

Bell K (1986) School accidents. *Health Bulletin*, **44**:2.
Health and Safety Executive (1974) *A Guide to the Health and Safety at Work Act 1974.* HS(II)6. London: HMSO.

Chapter 14
Child Abuse
Donna Mead   J R Sibert

When, in the 1950s, Kempe first drew the world's attention to child abuse it was greeted with some incredulity that parents could injure their children. Historically, however, this should not have been so surprising. Child abuse is as old as civilisation itself. Murder, maiming, wilful neglect, starvation, exploitation and abandonment of society's young have been reported throughout the ages: in Neolithic times some children were murdered by their parents for superstitious reasons. Actions such as this have been sanctioned by law, religion or by turning a blind eye; for example, there is evidence that harsh discipline was acceptable in biblical times: 'He that spares the rod spoils the child' (Proverbs XII:24). In Anglo-Saxon times it was thought better to kill Friday's child than to allow him to grow up in a life of misfortune, and in the mediaeval period, few children, of whatever background, escaped frequent beatings. It was common practice for poverty-stricken Georgian parents to abandon unwanted infants in the streets or to kill them and drop their bodies in dung heaps to avoid funeral expenses. In certain cultures children are mutilated by male and female circumcision, foot-binding and by the breaking of limbs to turn them into good beggars.

During Victorian times, however, the works of Christian men such as Lord Shaftesbury and Dr Barnardo created an awareness of the plight of many children in England and Wales, and in 1844 the National Society for the Prevention of Cruelty to Children (NSPCC) was formed. Despite these good works, the children of the Victorian era were cruelly abused. Somerset Maugham's *Lisa of Lambeth* shows the degradation of children in an inner city area at the turn of the century, in some ways reminiscent of the Third World today, with large families and high infant mortality being common.

The improvement of child care in the twentieth century anaesthetised people to child abuse, and the term "battered baby syndrome" shocked the world. Since the 1950s we have learnt much more about non-accidental injury (NAI), and we are much better at recognising the problem and dealing with it. It must be remembered, however, that child abuse has an appreciable mortality and morbidity and, therefore, needs to be dealt with with care, sympathy and expertise, just as, say, one would deal with children with cancer.

It is now recognised that the deliberate infliction of physical injury upon children is but one aspect of the total spectrum of child abuse, which includes emotional abuse, sexual abuse, non-accidental poisoning, Munchausen's Syndrome by Proxy, and neglect, including nutritional deprivation. These abuses may be present singly or, more commonly, in combination.

A typical example illustrates the problem. A second child of parents whose first child had thrived spent six weeks in the special care baby unit because he was born preterm. Having brought him home, his mother never really related to him and left him upstairs without feeding or playing with him. He was finally admitted to hospital when 13 months old, grossly wasted and withdrawn and with numerous bruises on his face and body.

Failure to bond may be associated with subsequent abuse. Staff working in maternity wards and special care baby units are now aware of this risk and take steps to avoid it. Nevertheless, this example serves to illustrate the combination of physical abuse, neglect and emotional abuse that can occur. Fortunately, the child concerned has now been adopted and is developing normally.

Combinations of types of abuse are also found in families. In one family, a girl of eight was subjected to sexual fondling by her father, a boy of six was physically abused by him, and a girl of two, who had been neglected, presented with failure to thrive.

Since the introduction of child abuse procedures it is possible to gain a more accurate idea of how many children are abused. The NSPCC estimate that 4699 children were physically abused in 1977 – of these, 822 were fatally or seriously injured. In 1982 the number of children physically abused had risen to 6388. However, of these, only 647 fell into the category of fatally or seriously injured, which may be the result of improved techniques for dealing with child abuse. Death rates are difficult to estimate. However, NSPCC statistics suggest that in England and Wales one child a week dies from child abuse.

Major psychiatric disturbance in the parents is unusual in most forms of child abuse. The results of several studies suggest that immature personality and a history of violence in early life are contributing factors. It is often the case that abusing parents were subjected to such abuse when they were young. Parents often have unrealistic expectations of the abilities of their children, for example in expecting a six-month-old child to be potty trained.

The results of epidemiological studies, however, are such that objective data to aid prediction of which children are likely to be abused are now available, as this type of family needs special consideration from the community medical services and, in particular, from the health visitor.

Physical Abuse

The physically abused child is the one most likely to be brought to the Accident and Emergency Department. It is now accepted that a combination of factors is usually involved in injuries that involve physical abuse, and Kempe and Kempe (1978) suggest that the parents' problems, the child, and the crisis are the aspects of most significance (Figure 14.1).

Murphy et al (1981) further examined the proposals of Kempe and Kempe, and it would appear that there is general agreement about the nature of these three aspects.

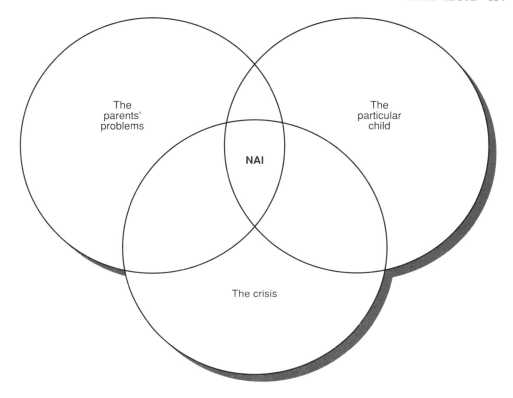

Figure 14.1 Factors involved in physical abuse

The Parents' Problems

These may be many and include:

1. Deprivation during the parents' own upbringing.
2. Unemployment.
3. Ill health.
4. Youth and immaturity, leading to inadequacy.
5. Single parenting.
6. Marital problems – e.g. forced marriage, violence.
7. Low intelligence.
8. Drug or alcohol dependency.
9. Frequent pregnancies, exhaustion or depression.
10. Aggressive or criminal tendencies.
11. Lack of family support.
12. Unreal expectations of the child.
13. Inadequate home and environmental conditions.

The Child

1. Often the result of an unwanted pregnancy.
2. Difficult pregnancy and/or labour.
3. Preterm or small-for-dates baby, resulting in prolonged separation from the mother and difficulty in bonding.
4. Neonatal illness.
5. Previous loss of a child of the same sex.
6. 'Wrong sex' child.
7. Hyperactive child, demanding much attention.
8. Child just different from the rest of the family.
9. Handicapped or slow-to-learn child.

The Crisis

This is the precipitating factor that results in the child being attacked by parents. The event may be something major, such as redundancy or news of another pregnancy. Alternatively, it may be a minor event such as the milk boiling over.

The Child's Injuries

The child's injuries may involve bruising of the face and head, burns and scalds, intracranial injuries, internal injuries and eye injuries, including retinal haemorrhage.

Bruises and Abrasions These are found on the normal, healthy child, particularly on the shins and forehead, and should not be viewed with suspicion unless associated with other injuries that are unusually severe, in abnormal positions (e.g. behind the ears or on the buttocks), or that are multiple and cannot be explained by a single accident. The exception to these conditions is the infant under 1 year of age in whom it is unusual to see bruises and where, therefore, the parents' account of how the injury occurred is of particular importance. An explanation such as 'the baby banged herself against the cot bars' should be considered with careful regard to the infant's stage of motor development.

It is unusual for a child to have grazes or bruises around the genital area, and any such injuries should arouse concern. Injuries to the soft tissues inside the mouth or a torn frenulum may have been caused by a feeding bottle being forced in, or by a blow. The soft tissues around the eye and face would normally be protected by the orbit and cheekbone. Bruising or petechial haemorrhages to the pinna of the ear may be caused by pinching, pin pricks or blows.

Figure 14.2 shows bruising on the face of a toddler, which was also evident behind the pinna and was due to a blow to the head. The child also suffered emotional abuse and neglect. In Figure 14.3 the bruising has been caused by a slap to the child's face – hand marks are clearly visible. As most adults are right-handed, such injuries are often on the left side of the child's face.

Bruises and abrasions caused non-accidentally can often be identified by their

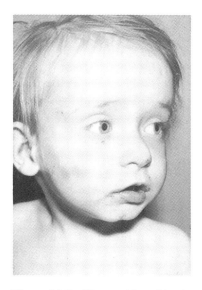

Figure 14.2 Non-accidental bruising to the face of a toddler

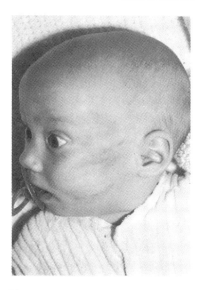

Figure 14.3 Bruising caused by a slap to the face

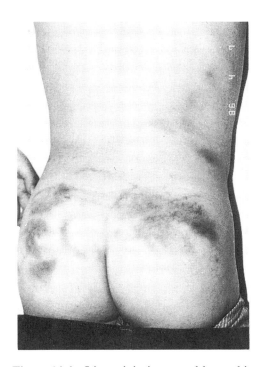

Figure 14.4 Linear injuries caused by a whip

appearance. Bruises caused by a belt, chain or cane can cause linear marks (Figure 14.4). Bruises caused by an acceleration or deceleration impact are generally accompanied by swollen tissue as well as bruising; these are often accidental. Bruises caused by compression, such as by finger pressure, however, are not associated with such swelling and are less likely to be accidental.

Bruises in a 'finger-tip' arrangement around the sides of the head or jaw are most likely to be caused by shaking the child. Bites can often be identified by dental impressions of the suspected abuser being matched to the injury. Bites appear as two half-moon shaped bruises opposite each other.

Coagulation disorders such as haemophilia need to be excluded in all cases of bruising thought to be due to abuse.

Burns and Scalds   Burns and scalds inflicted deliberately differ considerably from those caused accidentally. The 'dunking injury' is evidence of scalding deliberately inflicted, often as punishment upon the child who has wet or soiled his pants. It occurs when the child is deliberately dipped into or held in hot water. The scalds have a clear demarcation line or high-water mark, which may be seen on the feet, the buttocks or both. In the case of accidental injury, splash scalds are to be seen where the child has jumped into and scrambled out of hot water and so splashed drops onto other parts of his body. Splash scalds are not generally seen following dunking injuries.

Cigarette burns inflicted deliberately are circular and penetrate the skin. Accidental burns with a cigarette cause injuries that are usually minor and do not blister: the lesion may be linear where the child has brushed past the hot tip, rather than the perfect circle that results when the tip of the cigarette is held against the flesh.

Burns caused by holding a child over a fire to burn the buttocks produces a large area of erythema and blistering, which usually extends from thighs to lower back. This type of injury could not have been caused accidentally because the pain engendered by the heat would have caused the child to move long before the burn occurred. Figure 14.5 shows linear burn marks caused by holding the child's leg against the bars of an electric fire. This injury is another example of one inflicted as a punishment for wetting pants.

Fractures   Fractures may be seen as part of severe child abuse. Babies may sustain multiple rib fractures from being squeezed. Spiral fractures, particularly of the arm, may be caused by twisting a limb. Metaphyseal fractures of long bones should also be considered to be due to child abuse in young children and are caused by wrenching injuries. Fractured clavicles and skull fractures are sometimes caused in a non-accidental way. All children under two and many sustain multiple rib fractures from being squeezed. Spiral fractures particularly of the arm may be caused by twisting a limb. Metaphyseal fractures of long healed fractures demonstrating previous episodes of abuse: the X-rays may not demonstrate new fractures, however, which will only be shown up in children under two years of age, by an isotope bone scan.

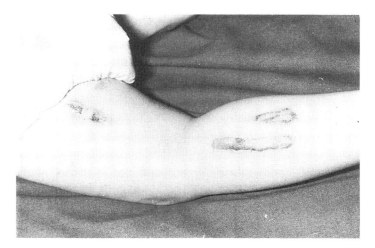

Figure 14.5 Linear burns from an electric fire

Intracranial Injuries Intracranial injuries account for the highest percentage of deaths from non-accidental injury but rarely, if ever, occur accidentally in the infant. They can be caused by acceleration, where a moving object such as a fist causes a blow to the head, or by deceleration, where the head is moved through the air and brought to rest against an immovable object, for example, in swinging the child's head against a wall while holding him by the ankles.

In the whiplash injury the child is held by the trunk and shaken vigorously; the head reverberates, rupturing small blood vessels in the subdural space, and a subdural haematoma accumulates, which can lead to brain damage and/or death. This is a most dangerous form of child abuse, but some parents believe it is an acceptable form of punishment: 'I never hit my child. I only shake her when she is naughty.' In injuries of this nature there is no outward sign, and the child is usually brought to the Accident and Emergency Department because he has the usual symptoms of head injury, for example progressive drowsiness, together with clinical signs such as unequal pupils.

Internal Injuries Internal injuries are the second most common cause of death after cranial injury. Again, such an injury may not be obvious and there may be no external signs. The soft abdomen of the infant is lacking in muscle and, as such, does not tighten up to withstand the blow; this allows maximum internal damage to be caused. The most common injuries are perforation of the small intestine and damage to the kidney. Physical signs may include an increasing abdominal girth or haematuria. Traumatic haemopericardium, haemothorax and traumatic pancreatitis are also known to result from non-accidental injury.

Traumatic Alopecia Some children may have been swung around or pulled by the hair, thus appearing to have partial alopecia.

Manifestation of a Situation of Physical Abuse

When a child has been physically abused the parents may delay for hours or days before seeking medical attention. Hospital attendance may be sought only when a head-injured child loses consciousness, or shock occurs following an internal injury or burn. Any delay in presentation should arouse suspicion and warrants further investigation.

Emotional Abuse

Emotionally neglected children may be ignored and left alone without stimulus for long periods. These children do not thrive, despite having an adequate food intake, and may have typical, cold, red extremities due to autonomic disturbance, which results in vascular stasis. Older children may be subjected to constant teasing and be forced to perform degrading acts; they may be prevented from going to school for no reason.

Emotionally abused children, particularly toddlers, may have retarded mental development. In babies the smiling and motor milestones, such as sitting, may be delayed, but more typical is speech delay in older children. One example is the child of a single, educationally subnormal mother, who when admitted to hospital had little recognisable speech: one month later, his speech was within normal limits. Such children need a full developmental assessment and may need special educational help when removed from their parents.

Recognition of emotional abuse can be difficult, and it is often only perceived when physical abuse brings it to attention. Indeed, emotional abuse may be the most damaging form of abuse to a child in the long term, and it is increasingly being recognised that these two forms of abuse often appear together. Generally, severe, emotional deprivation results in a child who is unable to give love or show emotion, a child with 'frozen watchfulness', one who has not been stimulated and who may well have been told 'Mummy doesn't love you'.

Sexual Abuse

Sexual abuse has only recently become recognised as a major problem. The whole issue has recently been fully investigated and published in the report of the enquiry into child abuse in Cleveland by Lord Justice Butler-Sloss (DHSS, 1987).

This report was issued in conjunction with two publications from the Department of Health and Social Security: *Child Protection: Guidance for Senior Nurses, Health Visitors and Midwives* (DHSS, 1988a), prepared by the Standing Midwifery Advisory Committee, and *The Diagnosis of Child Sexual Abuse: Guidance for Doctors* (DHSS, 1988b) by the Standing Medical Advisory Committee.

Most commonly, sexual abuse is incestuous, perpetrated by the child's father or stepfather (75 per cent of cases), but brother and sister, uncle and niece and mother and son incestuous relationships are less frequently encountered.

Information on sexual abuse is difficult to come by, as the causes are often hidden. It is a myth, however, that it only occurs in isolated or primitive societies, and what research there is suggests that all classes of people may be involved. It is also a myth that only post-pubertal girls are involved, for it has been suggested that the median age for starting an incestuous relationship is 9–10 years.

Although sexual abuse is more common in girls than in boys, the diagnosis should be suspected in both sexes. This is illustrated in the case of a nine-year-old boy who presented with non-organic abdominal pain. His stool contained *Trichomonas vaginalis* and it was later found that he had been sexually abused by his stepfather.

Sexual abuse is one of the most difficult forms of child abuse to detect. Detection, however, is absolutely necessary because there is no doubt that these relationships are deeply damaging to those involved, as shown in evidence from incest survivors. The offspring of relationships between first-degree relatives are much more likely to have congenital malformations and genetic recessive disorders than are those of unrelated parents.

For these reasons it is of utmost importance that those professionals who are involved in any way with the care of children are aware of the tell-tale signs of sexual abuse. The following signs and symptoms are based on material from a Ciba Foundation Study Group (Porter, 1984) and are reproduced with kind permission.

Signs and Symptoms of Sexual Abuse

Physical   In the rectal and genital area:

1. Bruises, scratches or other injuries, often very minor, not consistent with accidental injury.
2. Itching, soreness, discharge or unexplained bleeding.
3. Foreign bodies in the urethra, bladder, vagina or anal canal.
4. Abnormal dilatation of the urethra, anus or vaginal opening.
5. Pain on micturition.
6. Signs of sexually transmitted infections.
7. Semen in the vagina or anus or on the external genitalia.
8. Swelling of the labia.

General:

1. Bruises, scratches, bite marks or other injuries to breasts, buttocks, lower abdomen or thighs.
2. Difficulty in walking or sitting.
3. Torn, stained or bloody underclothes, or evidence of clothing having been removed and replaced (e.g. vest inside out).
4. Semen on skin or clothes.
5. Pregnancy in teenagers, especially where the identity of the father is vague or secret.
6. Recurrent urinary infections.
7. Psychosomatic features, such as recurrent abdominal pain or headache.

Behavioural Indications
Sexual:

1. A child who hints at sexual activity through words, play or drawings, or who hints at the presence of severe family conflict, family secrets or puzzling and/or uncomfortable things at home, but who seem fearful of outside intervention. (Note: Sex-education classes may lead some children suddenly to question what has been happening to them for years.)
2. A child with an excessive preoccupation with sexual matters and detailed precocious knowledge of adult sexual behaviour; one who repeatedly engages in age-inappropriate sexual play with peers, toys or himself; one who is sexually provocative or seductive with adults. This premature sexualisation of behaviour may lead to further sexual abuse.
3. Requests for information about contraception are rare but may be a cry for help.

General:

1. Sudden change in mood or behaviour, including regressive behaviour.
2. Sudden onset of wetting, day or night; prolonged bedwetting.
3. Changes in eating patterns, such as loss of appetite, faddiness or excessive preoccupation with food.
4. Loss of self-esteem and desire to make self unattractive; depression; frozen responses.
5. Lack of trust in familiar adults or marked fear of men (especially in female children who have been abused under threat or with force).
6. Pseudomature or overly compliant behaviour (often masking distress and anger).
7. Disobedient, aggressive, attention-seeking or restless, aimless behaviour with poor concentration.
8. Social isolation, with long-standing or sudden poor peer relationships: the child withdraws, plays alone and is often in a fantasy world.
9. Severe sleep disturbances, with fears, phobias, vivid dreams or nightmares, sometimes with an overt or veiled sexual content.
10. Inappropriate displays of affection between fathers and daughters; also jealous, possessive fathers who try to accompany their daughters everywhere and appear overconcerned or overinvolved with them.
11. Young teenagers who present with:

    - hysterical attacks;
    - self-mutilation;
    - suicide attempts (e.g. overdoses in adolescence);
    - persistent attempts to run away from home;
    - intensive sexual acting out, including promiscuity and, in some cases, prostitution.

The symptoms listed above should always be considered together with the physical signs as any behavioural change may be due to problems other than sexual abuse.

In school:

1. Poor peer-group relationships and inability to make friends.
2. Inability to concentrate, learning difficulties or a sudden drop in school performance. (For some sexually abused children, however, school may be a haven: the only place where they are allowed to function as a child. They may arrive early, be reluctant to leave and generally perform well.)
3. Marked reluctance to participate in phyical activities or to change clothes for PE, games, swimming, etc.
4. Regular avoidance and marked fear of school medical examinations.

Parents' behaviour:

This needs to be considered within the context that confronts the professional dealing with cases of suspected sexual abuse. Paradoxically, a father who appears overly concerned about his child is sometimes involved in child abuse of this nature. Detection is often made all the more difficult when the mother supports her partner or appears to distance herself from the situation, even though she may be aware of what is happening to her child or children.

Summary

There are no physical signs at the present time that can be regarded as uniquely diagnostic of child sexual abuse. The question of dilatation of the anus has been one of controversy. There may not be any abnormal physical signs detected around the anus, or there may be reddening and bruising present. Anal tone should be noted and the anus may dilate when the buttocks are parted. This physical sign is not conclusive of sexual abuse, but it should increase the level of suspicion.

It should be remembered that all the above signs and symptoms are 'indicators' and not proof of sexual abuse, and that if any of them are encountered, they must be considered in the context of the whole child and his family. This is important not only to avoid a false diagnosis but also to ensure that sufficient evidence exists to confirm actual child sexual abuse.

Non-accidental Poisoning

Non-accidental poisoning is often another symptom of stress within the home. The child is subjected to inappropriate drug administration, and it is fairly common to discover children who have been given their parents' anti-depressants or sedatives. In such instances it is often the case that the parents are unable to cope with a normal, lively child.

At the other end of this particular spectrum of child abuse, one finds children who are denied drugs when treatment is required for a medical condition. In such instances the parents withhold treatment so that the child becomes symptomatic and is admitted to hospital. An example of this situation is the young unmarried mother of a child with congenital heart disease. The child is regularly brought to the Accident and Emergency Department on a Friday night with cardiac symptoms, and is inevitably admitted to the ward because her mother denies withholding the child's treatment. Having found a 'free' babysitter the mother disappears for the weekend. The child is investigated but no new abnormality is detected, her usual medication is given and she responds well.

Munchausen Syndrome by Proxy

This form of child abuse is also referred to as Polle's Syndrome or Meadow's Syndrome. It involves the fabrication of symptoms in otherwise healthy children such that medical attention for the child and continued hospitalisation are achieved. Examples include:

1.   Adding salt to feeds, resulting in a state of dehydration.
2.   Adding sugar, or blood from a finger prick, to urine.

The result of such actions by the parents may be that the child has to undergo unnecesary and unpleasant investigations.

The parents in these cases are usually grossly disturbed and often have some medical, nursing or first aid knowledge. This condition can be dangerous: Meadow (1977) described the case of a child who had recurrent illnesses associated with urinary tract infections. The child was prescribed several courses of antibiotics, was admitted to hospital on 12 occasions and was subjected to a variety of investigations, including intravenous urograms and cystograms. The true situation was that the mother ws adding her menstrual blood to the child's urine.

Neglect

Neglect often manifests itself as nutritional deprivation: in such cases the child will present with a diagnosis of failure to thrive. This may be due to an inadequate food intake, which is occasionally the result of the parents insisting that their children follow rigid dietary fads such as veganism or macrobiotics. The parents are usually unaware that such diets are inadequate and do not satisfy the needs of a developing child. Emotional neglect, however, can also reduce growth. This is thought to be mediated by low growth hormone production.

Whether neglect is due to nutritional or emotional deprivation, the child will appear clinically to be thin and, possibly, pot-bellied. Following admission to hospital, weight gain occurs without any organic cause being found for the failure to thrive. A typical manifestation of this form of abuse is that on returning home the child once more loses weight. Neglected children may be ravenously hungry when in hospital, sometimes to the extent that they steal food from other children.

Napkin dermatitis is commonly found in neglected children (Figure 14.6). Napkin rash appears as small, 'punched out' ulcers about 0.5 cm in diameter. This is due to infrequent or non-changing of nappies.

While not exclusively the result of neglect, scabies, impetigo and head lice are often found in such children. Similarly, neglected children are often dirty, but it should be remembered, however, that dirt by itself is not a sign of neglect.

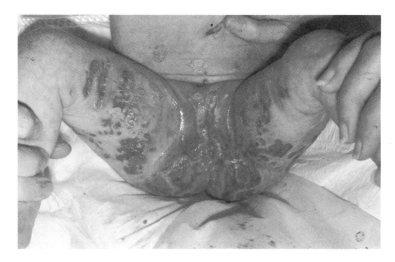

Figure 14.6 Severe napkin dermatitis with punched-out ulcers

The Diagnosis of Child Abuse

The diagnosis of child abuse can sometimes be very difficult, and it may be hard to steer a course between falsely accusing innocent parents and failing to recognise and deal with a child at risk. When in doubt, therefore, it is essential that advice is obtained from a more experienced colleague, if necessary through the local child abuse procedure.

It has already been demonstrated that the diagnosis of physical abuse is possible from the history of the accident. Sometimes, the injuries do not fit the explanation given. Figure 14.7 is an example of a bone scan in a child who was suspected of being abused but whose skeletal survey was normal. The scan shows increased uptake of isotope under the periosteum of the right tibia, which was caused by a fracture and its subsequent bleeding. The parents' explanation was that the child twisted his foot in the cot, but this is not compatible with the child's injuries. All children under two years of age who are suspected of being abused should have initial X-rays followed by a bone scan.

There may be a delay in presenting the child for medical attention, and the child may be presented to several different Accident and Emergency Departments. Recurring injuries should raise the suspicion of child abuse, but it should be remembered that the same social factors that predispose children to child abuse also predispose them to accidents. The presence of a child protection register in the Accident and Emergency Department may make the diagnosis of non-accidental injury easier. This register used to be known as the 'at risk' register. As the information held on the register is concerned primarily with future protection rather than post-abuse action, it was recommended that the register be renamed the Child Protection Register (DHSS, 1988).

Care should be taken to exclude clotting disorders such as haemophilia in cases of possible non-accidental injury: this can be done by performing a blood coagulation screen in all cases of bruising. With fractures, the rare possibility of

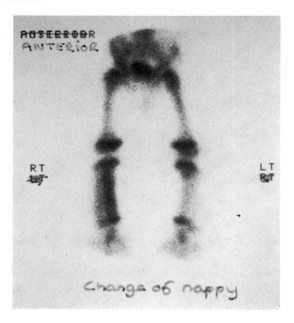

Figure 14.7 A bone scan in a child suspected of having been abused

a bone dysplasia such as osteogenesis imperfecta should be borne in mind. Unexplained bone fractures and multiple rib fractures in infants are most suggestive of non-accidental injury, even without other evidence of abuse.

The diagnosis of neglect may be more difficult and organic disease must be excluded; however, if the evidence is clear, unnecessary investigations such as jejunal biopsy should not be performed. If the problem is failure to thrive, the child should gain weight in hospital and may be ravenously hungry. If the child is returned home, the weight gain will not continue.

The diagnosis of emotional abuse is not easy but should be considered in a withdrawn child, particularly one with retarded developmental milestones. In younger children, red extremities may provide a clue. Often however, emotional abuse is only recognised when physical abuse brings it to attention, or when the school reports behavioural disturbances.

Similarly, the diagnosis of sexual abuse is not easy (see also section on sexual abuse above). The history, with information from both child and relatives, can be critical. Physical evidence such as that already described should be sought. This may need the special expertise of a police surgeon. When possible a woman police surgeon should perform the examination. At present, it is common practice for sexually abused children to be examined at the police station. This is not to be recommended because it can result in the child thinking that he or she, too, is in some way responsible for what has happened. Increasingly, police divisions have an arrangement with the district general hospital for a room to be set aside for this purpose. It is hoped that this trend will continue.

The Law and Child Abuse

Until 1991, when the Children Act (1989) will be implemented, the legal aspects of child care are generally under the Children and Young Persons Act 1969. The new Children Act will change a number of aspects of law regarding child care, particularly regarding Local Authority support for children and families in care and supervision.

Under the Children and Young Persons Act care proceedings need two stages: proof and disposition. The conditions of proof are that the child's development is being avoidably prevented or neglected, the child's health is being impaired or neglected or the child is being ill treated. There are also conditions for a Schedule 1 offender being in the same household, if the child is beyond control, if the child is in moral danger, if the child is not receiving full time education or if the child is guilty of an offence. The child should also be in need of care and control which he is unlikely to receive unless the court makes an order. The orders that are available to the court are: Care Order, Supervision Order, Recognisance, Hospital Order and Guardianship Order.

Under the Children Act 1989 Care Proceedings will be one stage and simpler. The Court may make a Care Order or a Supervision Order if the child concerned is suffering or is likely to suffer significant harm and that harm is attributable to the standard of care being below what could reasonably be expected or the child is beyond parental control.

An area which will particularly change will be the question of the emergency protection of children. Under the Children and Young Persons Act children can be removed by a Place of Safety Order. These are made by application to a magistrate usually by an officer of the local social services department or by the NSPCC. Place of Safety Orders can last for up to 28 days before a further application needs to be made to the juvenile court. Place of Safety Orders lasting up to 48 hours can be made by the police.

Place of Safety Orders will be replaced by Emergency Protection Orders. The Court must be satisfied that there is reasonable cause to believe that the child is likely to suffer significant harm if he or she is not removed or there is reasonable cause to suspect that the child is suffering or is likely to suffer significant harm or that the access to the child is denied and is required as a matter of emergency. Emergency Protection Orders can only last for a maximum of eight days. The applicant can apply once for a further seven days. Emergency Protection Orders can be challenged after 72 hours. In addition to the Emergency Protection Order there is a new order, the Child Assessment Order, which is to enable the assessment of a child's health and welfare where concern exists but there is doubt whether emergency action is justified. Only the NSPCC or Local Authority can apply and the grounds are that the applicant believes the child is suffering or is likely to suffer significant harm and an assessment is unlikely to be allowed without an Order. At the present time is is difficult to know how major a part the Child Assessment Order will play in child protection.

In addition to the emergency protection of children the way that care proceedings are dealt with in different courts will change. The majority of cases are now dealt with by the Magistrates Court. At the present time a number of judges are being particularly trained in child care matters and if care proceedings are thought by the local Magistrates' clerk to be particularly complex they will be referred on to a judge in the County Court. At the moment complicated cases are often dealt with by the High Court making the child or children concerned Wards of Court. This will not be available to Local Authorities directly although complicated cases may be dealt with by the High Court by referral from lower courts.

In addition to care proceedings there is the quite separate question of criminal proceedings against the person or persons who have abused children. Charges may be brought for actual bodily harm, grievous bodily harm, child neglect, incest etc. These cases are heard either in the Magistrates Court or in more serious cases the Crown Court.

Scottish Law

The law in Scotland is different from that in Englnd and Wales and involves its own Acts of Parliament. The major difference is that the police have only the function of investigating suspected criminal activity, whereas prosecution of suspected criminals in court is a function of the state-run 'Procurator Fiscal' system, which is staffed by trained lawyers as a full-time, salaried public service. The juvenile court is known as the Children's Panel and consists of one trained lawyer, or his deputy, called the Reporter, who is assisted in panel hearings by two lay voluntary assistants. The Children's Panel care proceedings are also held in private. The parents or the child have the right to have a friend or a legal representative present at the hearing.

Children at risk of abuse can be taken to a Place of Safety under the Social Work (Scotland) Act 1968 Section 37(2), as amended by the Children's Act 1975 Section 83(b). This is usually carried out by a social worker, police officer or a member of the Royal Scottish Society for the Prevention of Cruelty to Children (RSSPCC). The Place of Safety Order lasts for a maximum of 7 days and can be renewed by the Reporter for a further 21 days without a hearing, but any further extension has to be as a result of the Panel's decision. If the parents object to the grounds on which referral to the Children's Panel is made, the case must be heard, usually privately in chambers, by the Sheriff (the equivalent of the English County Court judge), who decides on the probability of proof either to dismiss the case or to refer it to the next session or hearing of the Children's Panel.

Children may be taken into the care of the local authority at any time the parents request under Section 15 of the Social Work (Scotland) Act 1968. If a child needs to be taken into the care of the local authority against the parents' wishes, the relevant statute is Section 16 of this Act. Section 16 orders are made by the Children's Panel, or by the Sheriff where facts are disputed.

As in England and Wales, if the magistrates find a case proven, they may ask for social enquiry reports, or make a Care Order.

The Role of the Nurse in Child Abuse

The nurse may be in a critical position in all stages of child abuse, from detection to final outcome. She may be the person who first suspects abuse; in particular, it is the health visitor in her unique position in family care who may see unusual and suspicious injuries that need investigation. Other nurses in the community, especially school nurses, may see lesions that could be non-accidental.

It is the responsibility of every nurse who is involved in any way with the care of children to be familiar with the local authority child abuse procedures. These are usually obtainable free of charge from the Director of Social Services' office and should be available in all children's wards and Accident and Emergency Departments, GP surgeries and health centres. Reference should also be made to the guidelines of the nurse's professional organisation. If a nurse becomes concerned about, and therefore to some extent responsible for, a child whose well-being is in question, such procedures will provide information which will enable her to:

1. get the child's care and physical and emotional condition assessed and treated;
2. prevent further and possibly more serious injury or suffering, which is often a very immediate threat;
3. ensure that, as far as possible, her intervention does no more harm to family structures and relationships, including those with professional workers, than is necessary to ensure the child's safety and future well-being;
4. conform with the law and professional standards of competence and conduct.

It is generally considered among the caring professions that these objectives can be met only with a multi-disciplinary approach of co-operation, teamwork and commitment to the protection and well-being of the child. The professions involved include doctors, nurses, social services staff, school teachers and police. The nurse, also, should be aware that basic to this system of multidisciplinary management are the following elements:

1. A system of case conferences at which information is shared, plans made for helping the child and family and responsibilities assigned. The case conference is discussed in detail later.
2. A central register of all suspected cases of child abuse, which is available to key workers 24 hours a day.
3. A system of keeping all cases under review while the child is considered to be at risk from further abuse.

Where child abuse is suspected, therefore, the nurse will, following discussion with her manager, report the matter to the local Social Services Department. Subsequently, the child will usually be brought to the hospital for assessment by a paediatrician.

Where nurses in an Accident and Emergency Department suspect child abuse, the paediatrician should be involved directly, and if non-accidental injury is confirmed, the Social Services Department will be contacted.

The interview with the paediatrician is a crucial one, as parents are often confused and aggressive. The senior nurse in the ward or area should usually be present. It is most important not to accuse parents of injuring their child, but rather to speak of injuries that are likely to be caused non-accidentally and of the need for medical and social investigation. It must be remembered that the true facts are not always easy to ascertain at the initial assessment. The interview and contact with the parents should be done as for any child entering the ward, concentrating first on basic medical and social information: this will have a calming effect on the situation.

If the social worker and the paediatrician agree that the injuries are probably non-accidental, the child abuse procedure should be followed. This usually means admission to hospital; if possible, this should be done voluntarily, but if there is a significant risk of the child being removed from the ward, a Place of Safety Order should be taken out by the Social Services Department. If the child is removed while on a Place of Safety Order, the local police should be contacted urgently.

Investigations, such as coagulation screening and a skeletal survey to exclude bony injury, are undertaken during the initial admission. Photographs are important for medico-legal purposes, as bruises may fade quickly. Social enquiries will be made during this time by the Social Services Department and, in severe cases, by the police.

The time spent in the ward while awaiting such enquiries and the case conference is often a difficult one for the nurse and parents. It would be easy to treat the family like any other admission, but this approach, although emotionally less taxing for the nursing staff, must be avoided. The nurse has to steer a course that ensures that other families in the ward are not made aware of the reason for admission, while allowing the parents concerned to feel that the nursing staff are aware of the sensitive nature of their situation and that they can be relied upon to preserve confidentiality and to deal with them honestly.

One of the most important skills in dealing with families in which a child has been abused is that of not inferring any value judgments during interactions with parents, and this skill has to be developed by all nurses. It is acknowledged that this is a difficult course to steer, so much so that some nurses cope by avoiding the family and the issues that arise. For example, whenever the parents raise queries, the nurse might respond by saying that these should be discussed with the medical staff. However, it is particularly important with families of this sort that the nurse–family relationship has its foundation in trust and honesty. Where this is not the case, scepticism of professionals results, which can be very damaging for the long-term management of the child and family.

A standard procedure is not recommended in these circumstances as each family will be unique in: the events preceding the incident, crisis or abuse, their coping mechanisms and the nature of the injuries inflicted. However, the principles of care are fundamental and include:

1. Making an assessment of the child's relationship with his parents/family. How do they react together? What is the pattern of visiting and staying?
2. Making an assessment of the child's behaviour generally. Is he hungry?

Does he relate well to other children on the ward? Does the child respond to cuddles and demonstrate any ability to show affection for dolls or soft toys? Does the child cower when a helping hand is stretched out, fearing it to be a violent assault. Should an accident such as spilling a glass of juice or wetting pants occur, is the child fearful of reprisals? What is the child's explanation for the injury?

3. Making an assessment of age-appropriate developmental milestones. For example, what is the stage of toilet training and is it appropriate to the child's age?

These assessments are particularly important if the child is said to have contributed to the accident through his or her own motor activities. To what extent are these activities consistent with the child's age and developmental level?

Continuous observation and assessment of the child and family constitute part of the nurse's unique contribution to caring for an abused child. Whereas the paediatrician will endeavour to be available for the parents to speak to, the nature of his job is such that he is peripatetic. The nurse, however, is the only one of the health-care professionals involved with the family at this time who is available for 24 hours a day. The nurse is also different from the paediatrician and social worker in that she does not have as much influence as they do when decisions over the child's future are being made at the case conference. Many parents realise this and the nurse, therefore, is perceived by them as being less threatening than the social worker and more readily available to talk to than the paediatrician. In order to facilitate a relationship in which parents will feel at ease when discussing the situation it is important that they feel able to relate to the nursing staff. To this end, care should be given by as few nurses as possible, so that such a relationship can develop between the nurse, the child and his family.

The parents should be involved throughout the period during which investigations are being carried out. Experience suggests that parents, who usually realise the wrong that has been done, will often misconstrue the power and intentions of professionals. It is not unknown for example for a parent to think that a child is being 'taken away', when, in fact, he is only being taken to the X-ray department.

It should be remembered that if photographs have to be taken, the age of the child and the position of the injuries may be the cause of extreme embarrassment. The problem is compounded if the child is old enough to be aware of the situation and the subsequent stigma and humiliation; certainly, the explanation given to the child would need to strike a balance between obtaining the child's co-operation and minimising embarrassment, while preserving respect between the child and parents. Children are notoriously good at turning such situations to their own advantage. If all respect for their parents is lost, an added strain is placed on any attempt to rejoin parent and child.

Clearly the situation represents an emotional 'land-mine' for the ward-based nurse. However, such situations can be dealt with successfully when all nursing actions have their foundation in the preservation of the dignity of both child and parent. However, it should be pointed out that if there is a risk of the child being injured again by visiting parents, they should be excluded from the wards. In practice, this rarely has to be done.

The Case Conference

The case conference is an important factor in the decision-making process that protects children who may have been subjected to abuse. The initial conference is normally held within 3 days of the start of the enquiry and is chaired by a senior social worker, usually a district officer. All the agencies involved are invited to send representatives. These usually include:

1. social workers;
2. the health visitor;
3. the paediatrician;
4. the police (usually a juvenile liaison officer);
5. the ward sister or her representative;
6. an NSPCC inspector.

The Role of the Nurse in Case Conferences

It is the belief of the Royal College of Nursing (*Child Abuse and the Nursing Professions*, 1984) that:

'there is complete unanimity amongst the nursing profession about the role and contribution of nursing staff in cases of suspected or actual child abuse. This includes the attendance of the nurse manager at case conferences, in addition to nurses of any speciality involved with the family.'

The Royal College of Nursing also states that:

'nursing staff, particularly health visitors, have a key role to play at case conferences because of their regular contact with families and their knowledge of the family background. Their contribution is vital and must continue.'

Tasks of a Case Conference

The following are the main tasks to be undertaken by every case conference:

1. To consider the purpose of the case conference.
2. To share and update information on the child, his family and his environment, and to identify any gaps in this information.
3. To share knowledge of, and concern about, the family and members of the household, including parental biographies and full family history.
4. To nominate a key worker, prime worker, or case manager.
5. In accordance with local policy, to decide whether or not parents should be invited to attend the case conference, and if they are, at what point they should be admitted.
6. To attempt to make a family assessment (including some estimate of the degree of risk to all the children).

7. To decide upon and record a detailed action plan of care, and to allocate responsibilities for its implementation, including the definition of the responsibility of the key worker and all other workers. This may include legal steps necessary to protect the safety of the child.
8. To ensure that the key worker is given multidisciplinary support and that adequate cover is provided in the event of sickness or absence.
9. To ensure that full copies of minutes are circulated to all professional staff at, and those invited but unable to attend, the case conference. Where necessary, minutes of a meeting should have appendices attached in which a recommended plan of action can be stated, e.g.:

   • the outcome of conference;
   • the appointment of the key worker;
   • the date of review.

10. To decide upon ongoing review procedures in relation to the case, and to consider the frequency of case reviews.
11. To decide whether or not the child's name should be entered in the Child Abuse Register, and to consider the criteria under which entry would be made.
12. To decide whether or not to inform the parents (and the child, if appropriate) of registration and its significance.
13. To decide who should undertake the task of informing the parents of registration and deregistration.
14. To decide upon a summary of recommendations, which should include those in point 9 above, and which may include legal action.
15. To offer opportunities for professionals to share concerns and possibly diffuse the anxiety that may be experienced by those most closely involved with the family in the special circumstances of child abuse.

When invited to attend a case conference, a nurse should notify the nurse manager immediately and endeavour to arrange a ward meeting so that the child and family can be discussed.

In preparing for the case conference, the nurse should carefully select the information to be included, distinguishing fact, hearsay and opinion in order to analyse the evidence and present an accurate professional opinion. Such an approach is also essential if the nurse is subsequently required to give evidence in court. In undertaking this, the nurse should ascertain what gaps in her information on the case exist and liaise with appropriate colleagues to ensure that a comprehensive, up-to-date report is presented.

Evidence that may be required from nursing staff can include areas such as feeding habits, how the child relates to his mother or to other children and whether or not the child is able to play in a way appropriate at his stage of development. Evidence relating to the injuries or bleeding times, for example, will be given by the medical staff.

In the case conference all participants objectively discuss their involvement with the family and their observation and assessment of the child and his family. It is to be hoped that a consensus decision regarding the action to be taken can be reached. However, it is ultimately the decision of the chairman and, therefore, the Social Services Department as to what happens. Anyone who disagrees strongly with the case conference decision should write to the Director of Social Services for the area, stating the reasons for disagreement and the course of preferred action. This is important for medicolegal reasons and in case a disaster such as the death of a child should occur. If the decision is to go for care proceedings, the child should be sent from the ward into temporary foster care as quickly as possible, although in some cases of neglect, a longer period in hospital will be needed for diagnostic purposes and to allow for further care.

Giving Evidence in Court

All visits to court are worrying, even to those experienced in giving evidence. However, the Juvenile Court is a private affair, without press or public present, and it should be remembered that magistrates are keen only to make the best decision in the interests of the child. In care proceedings three solicitors or barristers are usually present, one for the agency bringing the proceedings, another representing the child and the third representing the parents. Each may cross-examine a witness in turn, and the magistrate often also asks questions.

People find it distressing to have to give evidence against the parents in their presence. This is understandable; however, it is vital, in the child's interests, that evidence given should be accurate because the consequences of a wrong decision by the court may be to expose the child to further injury and neglect. Nevertheless, it is possible in many instances to go through this difficult experience and remain on friendly terms with the parents.

Giving evidence in criminal proceedings is more worrying in view of the public nature of such proceedings. However, the same rules apply: to give clear, concise evidence based on good notes and express opinions only on subjects that are directly related to nursing.

It is being increasingly recognised that considerable stress is encountered by professionals who work with families where children are at risk of abuse or have been abused. The Standing Nursing and Midwifery Advisory Committee (DHSS, 1988a) set out in their guidelines for senior nurses, health visitors and midwives that staff should be supported at all stages in the management of child abuse. In particular, the committee recommended that they should be supported at the case conference and in court, and also when the practitioner disagrees with the majority decision about the case.

The Future for the Abused Child

In the past many abused children placed in care languished in children's homes without real decisions being made about their future. This was damaging to the growth of the child's personality and resulted in the child himself being, in effect, punished for the abuse. It is now generally agreed that a decision about the child's future should be made quite soon after the Care Order, perhaps in about three months. If it is safe for the child to be reintroduced into the family, this should be done in a controlled way, perhaps with a contract between the Social Services Department and the parents. This is done under the protection of the Care Order, and if there are reasons for concern, the child can be removed to a place of safety. If it is unsafe for the child to be reintroduced, or if the reintroduction fails, the child may then be placed with long-term foster parents with a view, possibly, to adoption. This policy has resulted in the closure of many children's homes.

The medical, nursing and social services should keep in contact with abused children, at least in the short term, to monitor their care, growth and development.

Summary

It has to be remembered that at some time in their life most children suffer an accidental injury. While an awareness of the possibility of malicious injury is necessary, professionals should refrain from displaying overt suspicion until there is definite proof.

The aims of the caring professions should be to ensure that our children grow up and develop in a loving environment, with those children who have already been abused saved from further assault or neglect. In the long term the aim is to rehabilitate and reunite the family. While it is accepted that emergency intervention will always be necessary it should be the concern of those in the teaching and nursing professions, and those with a responsibility for health education, that society's future parents are informed of the needs of a developing infant and, therefore, prepared for the problems that arise in growing children.

One of the most encouraging aspects of the professional life of those involved with the care of children is seeing abused or neglected children blossoming in the care of foster parents, or sometimes with their own parents. This represents the optimistic side of non-accidental injury, and goes some way towards reconciling the long hours and heartache given to the care of such children.

References

Association of British Paediatric Nurses, Association of Nurse Administrators, Health Visitors Association, Royal College of Midwives, Royal College of Nursing and Society of Nurse Advisors (1984) *Child Abuse and the Nursing Professions*. A joint statement. London: ABPN, ANA, HVA, RCM, RCN and SNA.

Butler-Sloss (1988), *Report of the inquiry into child abuse in Cleveland (1987)*. London: HMSO.

Department of Health and Social Security, Standing Midwifery Advisory Committee (1988a) *Child Protection: Guidance for Senior Nurses, Health Visitors and Midwives*. London: HMSO.

Department of Health and Social Security, Standing Medical Advisory Committee (1988b) *The Diagnosis of Child Sexual Abuse: Guidance for Doctors*. London: HMSO.

Kempe R S and Kempe C H (1978) *Child Abuse*. London: Fontana Open Press.

Maugham S W (1897) *Lisa of Lambeth*. London: Heinemann.

Meadow R (1977) Munchausen syndrome by proxy: the hinterland of child abuse. *Lancet*, **ii**: 343–345.

Murphy J, Sibert J R, Jenkins J and Newcombe R (1981) Accidental poisoning preceding non-accidental injury (letter). *Archives of Diseases in Childhood*, **56**(1): 78–79.

Porter R (ed.) (1984) *Child Sexual Abuse within the Family*. London: Tavistock Publications.

Recommended Reading

Carver V (ed.) (1978) *Child Abuse: A Study Text*. Milton Keynes: The Open University Press.

Child Abuse and Neglect. Official publication of the International Society for Prevention of Child Abuse and Neglect. Oxford: Pergamon Press.

Jones D N (ed) (1982) *Understanding Child Abuse*. London: Hodder & Stoughton.

Lee C M (1978) *Child Abuse: A Reader and Source Book*. Milton Keynes: Open University Press.

Meadow R (1982) Munchausen syndrome by proxy. *Archives of Diseases in Childhood*, **57**: 92–98.

Meadow R (1985) Management of Munchausen syndrome by proxy. *Archives of Diseases in Childhood*, **60**: 385–393.

Sharman R L (1983) *Child Abuse: A Discussion Paper*. London: Council for the Training and Education of Health Visitors.

Useful Addresses

Incest Survivors Campaign
Hungerford House
Victoria Embankment
London WC2N 6NN

National Children's Bureau
8 Wakely Street
London EC1V 7QE

National Society for the Prevention of Cruelty to Children (NSPCC)
1 Riding House Street
London W1P 8AA

Chapter 15
The Role of the Nurse in Childhood Accident Prevention
Jean Gaffin

The contribution that individual nurses can make to child accident prevention depends on the setting in which they work. For some, advice on prevention might be part of the treatment process in, say, the Accident and Emergency Department (see Chapter 3) or on the paediatric ward (see Chapter 4). For those working in the community, the opportunities for preventive work arise as part of helping families with a wide range of health and allied problems (see Chapter 2).

The size and gravity of the problem of childhood accidents has been covered in Chapter 1. The reader will now understand that accidents are multicausal, and approaches to prevention must recognise this complexity. As discussed throughout the book, a logical approach to accidents is to look at the child, the agent that causes the accident and the environment, both physical and psychosocial. Preventive strategies must be discriminating and targeted towards preventing serious accidents, serious, that is, in terms of severity of injury or of affecting large numbers of children. Preventive strategies must analyse individual accident types. This strategic approach is well summarised by Avery (1987) who lists the following stages:

1. Collecting and analysing data.
2. Deciding against which accidents resources are to be directed.
3. Defining the most appropriate countermeasures.
4. Implementing the prevention programme.
5. Assessing the effectiveness of the programme.
6. Modifying the programme, if necessary, to go through the relevant stages again.

There are three major preventive strategies:

1. Education.

2.   Environmental change.
3.   Enforcement.

Education may be targeted at those looking after the baby and young child, and at the child. Equally important targets are those who might have care of the child (e.g. child minder or teacher), who make decisions that affect children (e.g. architect or planner) or whose behaviour can affect children (e.g. all drivers, who need to understand how children behave on the road, either as pedestrians or when playing outside). The medium of education can be one-to-one, in which the nurse has a particularly important role, or through publicity campaigns (including the use of the mass media).

Environmental change will cover the physical environment, although the psychosocial environment is also relevant, as earlier chapters have suggested. Changes in the environment can result from technological advance, as in the gradual replacement of open coal fires by central heating. Environmental changes can be much more effective in producing a safer environment than those dependent on human behaviour, e.g. individually persuading those with open fires to buy and fit effective fireguards. This point is linked with the debate about individual versus collective action: if the community takes action such as purifying the water supply, this is more effective than asking each individual to boil all drinking water.

Enforcement involves the introduction of rules or laws to try to prevent accidents; examples include ensuring that safety devices such as seatbelts are used and that consumer products are safe, e.g. regulations on the use of flameproof materials in children's nightdresses. Building regulations are also relevant, but the major problem here is that adults design and build for adults, rarely taking the special needs of children into account.

It is important to see these three strategies (education, environmental change and enforcement) as being complementary and not mutually exclusive. For example, the health visitor's role in suggesting to parents that they store dangerous household products out of the reach of young children is reinforced by the introduction by manufacturers of child resistant containers (CRCs) for their most dangerous products. Even if CRCs became mandatory, an educational role would remain, for example persuading people not to store products such as White Spirit in containers such as jam-jars.

Primary, Secondary and Tertiary Prevention

The aim in primary prevention is to ensure that the accident does not occur, as when the health visitor recommends a lockable drug cupboard or the shortening of a kettle flex. Secondary prevention is aimed at reducing the severity of injury produced by an accident, for example when the midwife ensures that a new mother leaves hospital with the baby suitably restrained in the car so that it is protected should a road traffic accident occur. Increased knowledge of first aid is another example of secondary prevention. Tertiary prevention is the prevention of long-term effects, physical and psychological; ways in which nurses can help are discussed earlier in this book.

A report on child accidents in the West Midlands (Hayes and Hanstead, 1982) suggests that however desirable it may be, it is not possible to prevent all accidents, in which case preventing the outcome – injury – should be the goal. The report sees accident and injury as different points in a chain of events, the intervention points of which are influencing accident prevention and working to prevent injuries and to minimise the effects of those injuries that do occur.

Preventing Child Accidents: Which Nurse and Where?

It is all too easy to see accidents as someone's fault, for example of the parent who momentarily turns away as baby crawls to the stairs or rolls off the bed, or the toddler who darts into the road. But were parents told about the link between the stages of development and the accident pattern likely to occur as these stages – not just informed, but actively encouraged to buy reins or a stair gate? It is important for advice and support to be non-judgmental and positive. This requires nurses to be well informed – and this is one of the major objectives of this book. Leaflets and posters are not enough: they need to be reinforced by nursing staff understanding the accident process and possible strategies for prevention, as well as realising how poverty or stress may prevent parents taking effective action to reduce the risks that their children face.

Earlier chapters have given many examples of ways in which nurses working in a variety of settings can become involved in accident prevention. Midwives, for example, have the opportunity of discussing with parents, as they plan for their new baby, the need for a safe home, covering a range of factors from the need for fire guards to the importance of keeping baby bouncers on the floor and not on a work surface.

The health visitor's role has been discussed in some detail in Chapter 2, in which the importance of her contribution to child accident prevention is made clear. Not least is her regular contact: seeing all babies and families, and continuing to see them at home, surgery or clinic. It is to be hoped that the Health Education Authority study on the health visitor and child accident prevention (Laidman, 1987) will lead to the development of support materials for health visitors as well as to a greater emphasis on accident prevention during their training.

Laidman would like to see liaison health visitors in all hospital Accident and Emergency Departments. More than half of all hospitals appear to have one (BPA, 1984), and a report from Surrey (Surrey Area Health Authority, 1979) describes the success of one such scheme. Liaison between hospital and community staff improved; children who had accidents could be visited and appropriate advice given; and patterns of accidents within families could be shown and support or intervention offered.

Central collation and analysis of the information can be useful: the Surrey study gave as an example the realisation that the balcony design on one large council estate was responsible for a disproportionate number of accidents involving falls; as a result, the balconies were modified. This shows the importance of involving nurse managers in such schemes: it was the initial central analysis of accident report forms that enabled the problem to be identified.

One crucial aspect of the health visitor's role is to explain the link between child development and accidents; the rolling and crawling of the early months, followed closely by the peak of poisonings at 13–24 months and the dangers in the same period of scalding, especially from cups of hot tea. Parents often underestimate their child's stage of development – the ability to climb onto a chair placed below an open window, for example. The problem of overestimating ability is also important, especially with regard to child pedestrian accidents. Children may not be ready to cross the road alone until the age of 9, but parents often see younger children as ready to negotiate minor roads, despite the complexity of the decisions that must be made even for minor roads.

Nurses in Accident and Emergency Departments and wards will see most of the two million children each year who it is estimated attend Accident and Emergency Departments (Wells, 1981). One problem is the need to be sensitive to non-accidental injury, as discussed in Chapters 1 and 14. It may be difficult to discuss the implications of an accident when confronted by urgent treatment needs, as well as by the pain, grief and guilt that serious accidents create. But at follow-up appointments and in cases of minor injury, the nurse involved in treatment has a unique opportunity to discuss the context of the accident; this is dealt with in detail in Chapter 3.

The school is another important setting in which nurses work. As discussed in Chapter 14, school nurses can encourage teaching about safety by trying to make teachers aware of the scope for accident prevention in the classroom, in the playground and during sporting activities. School nurses may also come into contact with accidents that can result from peer-group pressure – being 'dared' to do something. One study of American children aged 10–14 years showed that 12 per cent had been involved in risky activities following dares (Lewis and Lewis, 1984). The authors suggest that peer-group pressure had been recognised by those teaching adolescents about resisting social pressures to smoke. Their findings may point to a factor that needs considering in relation to preventing accidental injury to older children.

Education

Jackson (1980) states that:

'the role of safety education in reducing accidents is at first sight an important one, and over the years vast sums of money have been spent in the production and distribution of safety education material and in educational programmes. Yet evidence of the effectiveness of all this in actually reducing the number of accidents is very scanty. This is not to say there is no effect, but merely to say that the relationship is difficult to prove. Education has to increase people's knowledge, alter their attitudes and, if possible, to change their practice, and unfortunately the three things – knowledge, attitudes and practice – do not necessarily change together.'

Safety campaigns, when launched, need to be more skilfully aimed; in particular, they should be geared to age. The parents of the exploring toddler need a different message (e.g. information about cooker guards, fire guards or stair gates) than do those of the impulsive school child. The school child and adolescent need to be taught directly, and also need environmental help, such as a barrier outside the school to stop them dashing straight out into the road. The careful monitoring of accidents, which may lead to the modification of balconies for example, as outlined above, is more effective than are posters about the danger of falls from balconies.

Several projects to evaluate health education campaigns have been carried out. Minchom et al (1984) in Cardiff aimed to test the assumption that health education directed at parents and children can reduce child accidents. A conventional campaign was carried out and monitored by looking at children attending the local Accident and Emergency Department. A slightly increased willingness to attend hospital for trivial injury suggested that the campaign lowered the threshold of parental anxiety. The authors concluded that changing the environment (e.g. by using safe surfaces in playgrounds) can be more effective than trying to educate the public to adjust to the environment.

Health visitors in Sweden use a check-list to guide them in looking for specific hazards relevant to the children visited and to make parents aware of the safety implications of each stage of development (Gustafson et al, 1979). This kind of education overlaps environmental change: education can modify the child's environment, e.g. by encouraging parents to push the kettle to the back of the work surface so that when children start to stand they cannot tug the kettle flex.

Particularly for the under fives, it is the education of parents that matters most. One of the most effective mass media campaigns of recent years has been the BBC television series 'Play it Safe', which was introduced by Jimmy Savile. Evaluation found that 59 per cent of the adult population saw at least one programme and it was backed up by the distribution of over two million copies of the *Play it Safe* booklet. Many local educational and promotional campaigns and research projects were linked to the films. One study (Colver et al, 1982) took place in a deprived inner city area and showed that of the families encouraged to watch the programme, only 9 per cent took action to make their home safe. More encouraging was the finding that 60 per cent of those families given specific advice about hazards in their home during a home visit made at least one change to make their home safer. The authors suggest that advice will be heeded by families most at risk if the advice is specific, detailed, relevant and given at a pre-arranged home visit. Such a critical approach to health education is preferable to the distribution of posters and leaflets without consideration of their effectiveness. Nevertheless, Williams and Sibert (1983) found that hospital admissions for serious accidents (burns and fractured femurs) did not reduce during the period of the 'Play it Safe' campaign.

Other relevant studies include one undertaken by Dershwitz (1977) in the USA to prevent household injuries: researchers visited and discussed home safety with a selected group of mothers who were asked to work their way through a booklet giving specific advice; they were telephoned to encourage continued participation. The home safety of this group, and a control group of mothers given no booklet, was assessed by visitors who did not know which group they were visiting. No difference between the hazards in the homes of the two groups was found.

Earlier research (Schlesinger, 1966) looked at the effectiveness of health education for parental groups in relation to the incidence of accidental injuries to young children. A middle-class New York suburb was divided into two groups: there were over 4000 children under seven years of age in each group. One set had group discussions, printed materials, newsletters, etc., and the other had nothing. There was no difference in the accident rates between the two groups over a period of three years during and after the experiment.

That health personnel do not take advantage of the opportunities that present themselves was shown in a study of 377 childhood accidents in Southampton (Cliff and Li, 1983): 72 per cent of respondents had received no information from a health-care professional about accident prevention.

Another important aspect of education involves ensuring that decision-makers are informed about the importance of childhood accidents and their role in preventing them. Another strategy for prevention is ensuring that accidents are on the agenda of agencies like the housing maintenance section of a local authority housing department or the committee responsible for playgrounds, so that accident prevention competes with other demands for a share of scarce resources. An example of the wide range of authorities responsible for certain accident hazards is shown in Table 15.1.

Environmental Change

The success stories in the history of accident prevention are in the area of environmental change, often backed up with the sanctions of enforcement. One such success story is that of the reduction of poisoning of children after the introduction of CRCs. Regulations concerning the safer packaging of analgesics were introduced in 1976. It has been shown (Sibert et al, 1981) that hospital admission for analgesic ingestion by children under five years of age fell from 3884 in 1974 to 990 in 1978. The authors point out that there was a reduction in other poisonings during the same period, suggesting a growing awareness of the poisoning as a result of the discussion about CRCs.

There was a similar debate prior to the introduction by manufacturers of CRCs for some household substances such as bleach. It was suggested (Craft et al, 1984) that it was unwise to package all household products in this way; CRCs should be restricted to substances such as turpentine, white spirit and caustic materials that caused serious symptoms. This paper showed the importance of careful examination of Accident & Emergency records for the development of specific preventive strategies; the records showed that 95.4 per cent of children recorded as having an episode of household product poisoning had no serious symptoms.

A Department of Trade (1980) study of prevention through product and environmental design suggested that paraffin heaters were the source of many fires before the British Standard was changed in 1955, but that no dangerous heaters were sold after that date, although older products would have been used for some years before being discarded. The authors point out that the less safe products would have been used by the lowest socioeconomic groups but that in the end they would eventually disappear. Nevertheless, the current economic

Table 15.1   Authorities responsible for minimising certain childhood accidents (From Avery, 1987. Reproduced by kind permission of CAPT and West Midlands RHA)

Hazard	Authority
RTAS	County engineers – Road Safety Officer, Police
Transport accidents (except RTAs)	Individual agent, e.g. British Railways Board
Houses	
Council	District Council Housing Department
Private	Individual owner
Poisons	
Drugs	Police, Drug Squad, Family Practitioner Committee
Household products	Ministry of Agriculture
Plants, Insects	Trading Standards Department
Fire	County Fire Service
Gas	Regional Gas Board
Electricity	
Domestic	(Regional) Electricity Authority
National grid	Central Electricity Generating Board
Building sites	Individual contractors, District Council
Industrial premises	Individual company
	Health and Safety Executive
Playgrounds (public)	District Council Planning Department or Amenities Department
Sports fields	
Private	None
School	Local Education Authority, individual school
Public Places (e.g. cinemas)	Individual owner
Shops	Local Authority Environmental Health Department
Canals	British Waterways Board
Swimming baths	
Public	District Council Amenities Department
Private	None
Rivers	(Regional) Water Authority
Beaches	District Council Amenities Department
Farms	Ministry of Agriculture
Firearms	Police
Animals	Ministry of Agriculture Divisional Veterinary Officer
	Local Authority Environmental Health Department

Special Note:
1. In most of these hazards the *individual owner/licensee* has personal responsibility to ensure that his facility/product is made as safe as is reasonably possible.
2. The Local Education Authority (LEA) has an overall responsibility to educate (parents and) children about all the hazards of the natural and man-made environment.

problems faced by many families with children may reverse improvements in a small but vulnerable number of families; for example household products may be kept in use, safety devices are not bought and cheaper and more hazardous means of heating are used. No accident prevention strategy can be successful when families lack the basic amenities, as, for example, do the homeless families living in bed-and-breakfast accommodation in London.

Recent design improvements include the development of softer surfaces for playgrounds, minimising the injuries when children fall from equipment and the increasing use of safety (i.e. toughened and laminated) glass.

The successful American accident prevention programme 'Children Can't Fly' (Spiegel, 1977) has been mentioned above. It was designed to reduce mortality and morbidity from falls from New York tenement block windows and included home visits, community education, a media campaign and the distribution of 16 000 free window guards. Falls and deaths in children under 15 were shown to have been reduced overall, and there were no falls reported at all from the windows fitted with guards.

Architects and designers are slowly becoming more sensitive to the needs of children and are avoiding such dangerous features as balconies with horizontal bars, easy access to garage roofs, glass doors at the bottom of staircases and cupboards placed above cooking stoves. The book *Child Safety and Housing* (CAPT, 1986) encourages safer design and planning in the same way as their pamphlet *Keep them Safe* (1986/7) encourages the purchase of safer consumer products.

The advantage of environmental over educational approaches to accident prevention is not merely that they can be shown to work but that the whole community benefits from such action. When glass is made safer, cycle lanes are developed or CRCs introduced we all benefit – rich or poor, young or old and whatever the degree of stress in our families.

Enforcement

The introduction of a law making it mandatory to wear seat belts in the front seats of cars is one of the most successful examples of legislation to prevent injuries, even if the number of accidents is not reduced. The Times reported on 30 April 1984 that hospitals were treating 20 per cent fewer car crash casualties, and that the number of accident victims requiring in-patient treatment had fallen by more than 35 per cent since the wearing of seat belts had become compulsory.

One major example of improvement from product change arises from regulations made in 1964 that laid down a higher standard of resistance to flame spread for children's nightclothes. The regulation was followed by a sharp reduction in child deaths from burning, although the move to central heating already mentioned is also relevant in this context.

Babies still die from scalds in baths despite displays of posters and constant exhortations to put the cold water in first. A mandatory lower temperature for hot water systems would reduce this risk and create a safer environment for the elderly as well as for children.

The major agency concerned with consumer safety legislation is the Consumer Safety Unit of the Department of Trade and Industry. The Unit is responsible for collecting and analysing statistics on home accidents: the Home Accident

Surveillance System. The Department is responsible for consumer safety legislation and has the power to ensure that dangerous products are not sold; such bans can be immediate, as was the case with scented erasers in 1984.

Conclusions

It is important to recognise the limitations of the extent to which accidents can be prevented. This is particularly true if we look beyond the physical environment discussed earlier and think of the social environment in which accidents occur. We may encourage the buying of cooker guards and help to make the built environment safer, but the relevance of overcrowding, stress and poverty should not be underestimated. Adult supervision in preventing accidents to the under-3s may be crucial, but the extent to which stress may make it difficult for the adult to supervise effectively needs to be recognised. Society is creating more stress: unemployment, complicated social security provisions, reduced expenditure on repairs to existing dwellings and the building of cheap accommodation to rent. All this will make it more difficult for nursing staff to advise families on prevention or to give accident prevention the priority it needs when viewed in the context of the mortality and morbidity rates of childhood accidents, as outlined in Chapter 1.

In Sweden one development is that of the appointment of child environment supervisors, with parents trained to identify and eliminate hazards. Child environment committees have been set up with representatives including child health centre nurses as well as teachers and social workers. All accidents are reported, and environment supervisors visit the sites to see what can be done to prevent a recurrence. An example of their success is the removal of delapidated cars. Other action includes increased use of helmets for child cyclists and, in one instance, a family rehoused from a dangerous flat. Overall, there is more advice given on accident prevention by nurses at child health centres in Sweden than in the UK (Avery, 1980). Is this attempt at accident prevention through community development a role that community nurses might wish to take on? Laidman has suggested an enhanced role for health visitors. This will succeed only if sufficient resources are allocated to make this possible.

The major changes to the social environment that could help to combat poverty, poor housing and unemployment may seem beyond the control of nurses, but as citizens and as health-care professionals they can encourage political arguments at both national and local level, perhaps by influencing policy-makers as well as patients to understand the underlying problems (Gaffin, 1981). Practical help is, nevertheless, still important, such as the introduction of an infant car seat loan scheme pioneered by the Fife Health Board. Perhaps mothers could also be encouraged to run a loan system for other safety devices. Community nurses who encourage such a system could be making a significant contribution to a safer environment, as Fife is doing in the case of safer car journeys.

Nurses can use their unique role in the community to communicate their concern for accident prevention and the strategies that can be realistically encouraged for specific target groups. Figure 15.1 shows a scheme for specific

It may be very worth while to consider carrying out a series of *special measures* relating to specific and well-defined accident problems. Where this is going to be done it is important to select the appropriate target group, highlight the particular problem and then work out in detail the specific remedies. A good example is *poisoning*, for which the following measures may prove beneficial:

The Problem

Target groups
1. Toddlers, especially boys aged 2–5 years
2. Teenagers, especially girls taking overdoses or boys and girls taking alcohol, solvents or hard drugs

Products involved
1. Medicines (70 per cent of cases), especially analgesics, sedatives and hypnotics
2. Household products (15 per cent of cases), especially bleach
3. Plants (5 per cent of cases), especially deadly nightshade and certain fungi (mushrooms)

The Remedies

for *Medicines*
1. Childproof medicine containers, especially for analgesics
2. Individual packaging of medicines
3. Lockable drug cabinets
4. Less widespread use of known toxic products, e.g. barbiturates
5. Medicines kept out of reach of children
6. Proper labelling of medicines
7. Avoidance of sweet-like medicines (e.g. Smartie-like iron tablets)
8. Collection of unused medicines
9. Public awareness campaigns

for *Household products*
1. Storage out of reach of children
2. Adequate labelling
3. Avoidance of manufacture of products resembling children's drinks or foods

for *Plants*
1. Avoid ingestion of known potentially toxic plants, e.g. deadly nightshade and some mushrooms

Note: *Very effective secondary prevention* for an accidental ingestion of most of these products (except for petroleum distillates, caustics, corrosives) is to keep available a single dose (5 ml) of ipecacuanha in order to induce vomiting

Figure 15.1 Special measures taken to combat particular poisoning risks (from Avery, 1987. Reproduced by kind permission of CAPT and West Midlands RHA)

measures in relation to just one accident type – poisoning.

If nurses view accident prevention seriously, take an interest in local accident patterns and encourage local action and national lobbying as well as being involved in realistic constructive, sympathetic advice, perhaps we may move further along the path to reducing mortality and morbidity from childhood accidents. We must always remember the need to be realistic and to recognise that the vast majority of childhood accidents result in minor injuries, which are unavoidable and a natural part of growing up. However, efforts must be made to prevent serious accidents. Nurses are listened to. They are aware of the hazards to children in the home and in the environment as well as of the cost to the family of accidents. Nurses should be prepared to give a little time in the hospital and the community to share this awareness of child development and local hazards with the adults and children they meet and care for.

References

Avery G (1987) *Childhood Accidents: An Action Plan*. West Midlands: Child Accident Prevention Trust and West Midlands RHA.

Avery J G (1980) The safety of children in cars. *The Practitioner*, **224**: 816–821.

British Paediatric Association (1984) *Joint Statement on Children's Attendances at Accident and Emergency Departments*. London: BPA.

Child Accident Prevention Trust (1986) *Child Safety and Housing*. London: Bedford Square Press.

Child Accident Prevention Trust (1986/7). *Keeping them Safe: A Guide to Child Safety Equipment*. London: CAPT.

Cliff K and Li H (1983) Children in danger: accidents in the home. *Nursing Mirror*, **156**(7): i-viii.

Colver A (1982) Promoting children's home safety. *British Medical Journal*, **285**: 1177–1179.

Craft A W, Lawson G R, Williams H and Sibert J R (1984) Accidental childhood poisoning with household products. *British Medical Journal*, **288**: 682.

Department of Trade (1980) *Personal Factors in Domestic Accidents: Prevention through Product and Environmental Design*. London: Consumer Safety Unit, Department of Trade.

Dershwitz R A (1977) Prevention of childhood household injuries: a controlled clinical trial. *American Journal of Public Health*, **67**: 1148–1155.

Gaffin J (1981) *The Nurse and the Welfare State*. Aylesbury: HM+M.

Gustafson L H, Hammarstram A, Linder K, Stjernberg E, Sundelin C and Thulin C (1979) Child-environment supervisors: a new strategy for prevention of childhood accidents. *Acta Paediatrica Scandinavica*, **275** (supp.):102–107.

Hayes H R M and Hanstead J K (1982) *A Report on Child Accident Prevention Studies in the West Midlands Region*. Birmingham: West Midlands Regional Health Authority.

Health Education Council and the Scottish Health Group, in association with the BBC (1981) *Play it Safe: A Guide to Preventing Children's Accidents*. London: HEC/SHEG.

Jackson H R (1980) Towards more effective prevention of child accidents. Paper presented to National Children's Bureau Seminar, London.

Laidman P (1987) *Health Visiting and Preventing Accidents to Children*, Research Report No. 12. London: Health Education Authority.

Lewis C E and Lewis M A (1984) Peer pressure and risk taking behaviours in children. *American Journal of Public Health*, **74**: 580–584.

Minchom P E, Sibert J R, Newcom R G (1984) Does health education prevent childhood accidents? *Postgraduate Medical Journal*. **60**: 260–262.

Schlesinger E R (1966) A controlled study of health education in accident prevention. *American Journal of Diseases in Childhood*, **111**:4.

Sibert J R, Maddocks G B and Brown B M (1981) Child resistant packaging and accidental child poisoning. *Lancet*, **2**: 289–290.

Spiegel C N (1977) 'Children can't fly': a program to prevent childhood morbidity and mortality from window falls. *American Journal of Public Health*, **67**: 1143–1147.

Surrey Area Health Authority (1979) Accident surveillance system. Paper presented to Health Visitors Association Conference, 1979.

Wells N (1981) *OHE Briefing: Accidents in Childhood*. London: Office of Health Economics.

Williams H and Sibert J R (1983) Medicine and the media. *British Medical Journal*, **286**: 189.

Further Reading

Child Accident Prevention Trust (1986) *Burn and Scald Accidents to Children*. London: Bedford Square Press.

Child Accident Prevention Trust (1986) *Keeping Safe*. London: Bedford Square Press.

Cliff K S (1984) *Accidents: Causes, Prevention and Services*. London: Croom Helm.

Constantinides P (1987) *The Management Response to Childhood Accidents: a Guide to Effective Use of NHS Information and Resources to Prevent Accidental Injuries in Childhood*. London: King's Fund Centre for Health Services Development.

Golding J (1986) Accidents. In: *From Birth to Five: A Study of the Health and Behaviour of Britain's 5-year-olds* Butler N R and Golding J (eds.). Oxford: Pergamon Press.

Kohler L and Jackson H (1987) *Traffic and Child Health*. Goteborg, Sweden: The Nordic School of Public Health.

Index